STARK CHOICES
A SURGEON'S STORY

STARK CHOICES
A SURGEON'S STORY

FROM PRAGUE TO LONDON AND BEYOND

JAROSLAV STARK

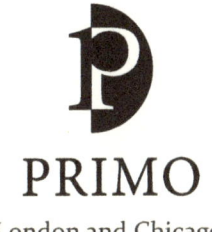

PRIMO

London and Chicago

Primo
An imprint of Peter Owen Publishers
81 Ridge Road
London N8 9NP

Copyright © Jaroslav Stark 2016

All rights reserved
No part of this publication may be reproduced in any form
or by any means without the written permission of the publisher

A catalogue record for this book
is available from the British Library

ISBN 978-0-9935327-0-2

Printed and bound in Great Britain by
CPI Group (UK) Ltd, Croydon, CR0 4YY

Typeset by Octavo Smith Publishing Services
www.octavosmith.com

CONTENTS

List of Illustrations	7
Prologue: Prague, 1968	9
1. Childhood, 1934–1945	15
2. Post-War Years, 1945–1947	21
3. Communist Takeover, 1948	24
4. Medical School, 1952–1958	30
5. Graduation and First Year of Medical Practice, 1958	34
6. Military Service, 1958–1959	37
7. Rychnov nad Kněžnou, 1959–1962	40
8. Prague, 1963–1965	47
9. London, 1965–1967	50
10. Back in Prague, 1968	57
11. London, 1968–1970	60
12. Boston, 1970–1971	66
13. Back in London, Early 1970s	72
14. London, 1973–1974	82
15. Lectures and Publications, 1975	93
16. Travels, 1979–1982, and a Visit to China	105
17. Icelandic Connection, 1981	119
18. The New Cardiac Wing, 1978–1987	121
19. My Books, 1979–1989	124
20. Further Trips and Lectures, 1983–1985	127
21. On Sabbatical, 1986–1987	137
22. Honorary Membership of the American Association for Thoracic Surgery, 1988	154
23. International Meetings and Congresses, 1989–1993	157
24. The Catching Up Trust and DAR, 1989–2000	161
25. The European Association for Cardio-Thoracic Surgery, 1987–2004	165
26. Worldwide Travel and the Glenn Lecture, 1994–1996	170
27. Database Conflicts, 1997–1998	178
28. The Bristol Inquiry, 1996–1998	181
29. The Bergamo School, Medicine and the Law	185
30. Family and Home Life	189
31. Patients and Their Families	194
32. Retirement	199
33. House Renovation and Further Holidays, 2008–2015	212

ILLUSTRATIONS

My mother, Jiřina Starková, and my father, Jaroslav Stark, in 1939
Me with my paternal grandfather, Jaroslav, at six months
Me in 1937, aged three, with my mother and six-month-old sister, Jiřina
On my rocking-horse, 1938
Me skiing in Radhošt, 1940
The family summer-house, built in 1939, in the village of Senohraby
With my sister Jiřina in Senohraby, 1941
Me as a sea scout, 1947
With my father in Senohraby, 1955
With Jiřina before her secondary-school ball, c. 1953
Olga (née Slugová) after her graduation ceremony, 1958
Olga and I are married in Prague, 1959
On our wedding day, 1959: Olga, my best friend Saša Kučera and I parody Stalin's monument
My first teacher, Dr Jaroslav Kudr, 1962
Professor Václav Kafka, head of the Department of Paediatric Surgery, University Hospital, Prague, 1964
David Waterson, my consultant at Great Ormond Street, 1969
Iain Aberdeen, a consultant at Great Ormond Street, late 1960s
Me in fancy dress at two Great Ormond Street parties
My son Jaroslav, Cambridge, 1979
The three Jaroslavs – my son, my father and me – Austria, 1983
Me negotiating the giant slalom during the annual 'Cardiac' skiing meeting in Courcheval, 1986
Me with Bill Williams in Toronto, late 1980s
My son Jaroslav and Kate (née Hardy) on their wedding day, 30 May 1987
Jaroslav's and Kate's wedding reception at Anson Road, Tufnell Park, London

I receive the gold medal at Charles University, Prague, 1998

Three pictures of a patient diagnosed with an inoperable transposition of the great arteries: as a four-year-old in 1975; seven years after the operation, playing basketball for the cardiac patients' team against the Harlem Globetrotters in London; with her boyfriend on holiday in Greece, aged thirty-six

In China, 2004: me dressed as a Chinese emperor in Beijing and with Sheelagh during the captain's reception on our Yangtze river cruise

Sheelagh and I, Machu Picchu, Peru, 2006

Sheelagh and I are married, 1 February 2011

Grandson Daniel with his mother Kate

Sheelagh and I in southern France, 2013

In 2014 I receive a silver medal from Charles University, Prague, and a gold medal from the Medical School in in the Karolinum

PROLOGUE
PRAGUE, 1968

It all started near Salzburg in August 1968. We were on holiday in Yugoslavia, camping on Veli Lošinj Island. It was an idyllic place – very different from our homeland, Czechoslovakia, with its tense political atmosphere. There it was anticipated that the Russians might invade at any time. We expected the worst, so we took our medical diplomas with us just in case we had to remain abroad.

On the campsite a few small items were stolen from our tent – a tin of frankfurters and Olga's cheap wristwatch – and we were very upset at the time. Yet, a few days later, after our return to Prague, we abandoned everything in our flat and left for England with one small suitcase. Somehow this didn't bother us. We were just relieved to get away.

Returning from Yugoslavia in our small Fiat 600 we camped in Salzkammergut near one of the lakes, but it started to snow, so we packed up the tent and drove straight home. We arrived at lunchtime on 20 August, and that night the so-called 'friendly armies' of the Warsaw Pact woke us up. We heard loud noise from the landing of Russian transporter planes; not long after this we became aware of Russian tanks rumbling along our streets.

Through tuning in to national radio we realized what was going on. On the pretext of assisting us against German counter-revolutionary forces the armies of the Warsaw Pact had invaded. Clearly Alexander Dubček's efforts to implement 'socialism with a human face' cut no ice with the Soviet leader Leonid Brezhnev.

Later on, in Britain, when I talked to my English friends I discovered they were under the impression that Dubček had introduced a number of reforms and that things in Czechoslovakia had changed considerably for the better under his leadership. They were not aware that the most significant reform that Dubček implemented during his short time as First Secretary of the Communist Party – the most powerful political position in Czechoslovakia –

was the abolition of censorship. But this was enough to provoke invasion. When the Russian papers and television claimed that there had been counter-revolution in Czechoslovakia supported by the German imperialists, the next day articles, signed by thousands of Škoda factory employees and workers from other large factories, appeared in the Czech press. They stated that the country was behind Dubček and that the Soviet allegations were 'bullshit'. This made Russian propaganda on this subject difficult to maintain. A cartoon lampooning this was published in the Czech *Literální noviny* (*Literary Gazette*), showing a car with President Svoboda and his minister of defence, Dzur. Svoboda is driving, and at the crossroads the Minister says, 'OK from the right. Tanks from the left!'

Czechoslovakia's geographical position meant that the Russians could not risk us leaving the Warsaw Pact. It would create a huge rift in its border against the West.

That morning I went to Prague University Children's Hospital where I worked as a cardiac surgeon. We expected casualties from all the fighting on the streets and readied ourselves to accept wounded civilians of all ages, although as a children's hospital the staff had to make a number of adjustments in order to take in adult patients. Just hours later I found myself travelling by ambulance to a Czech radio station that had put out a call for medical assistance to aid casualties there. It was a hair-raising drive – we passed a number of Russian tanks, one in flames, and had to make a detour to take a wounded civilian to hospital. In the end I spent three days in my department, with no opportunity to return home or even to communicate with my wife Olga, as my position at the hospital was not regarded as sufficiently senior for us to have been allocated a home phone. This was despite the fact that shortly before this I had spent two years in London learning the most up-to-date techniques involved in children's heart surgery and was the only member of the team with such experience.

Olga looked after our eight-year-old son Jaroslav while working in Smíchov, on the left bank of the river Vltava, as a paediatrician. Her surgery was on the other side of the river, so her journey from our apartment was somewhat fraught. With Russian tanks everywhere and with an eight-year-old child in the car it was a gruelling drive. After five days or so, our entire government, with President Svoboda at the helm, travelled to Moscow to negotiate with the Russian Politburo. We Czechs swiftly discovered that

PROLOGUE: PRAGUE, 1968

Dubček and three others had been arrested, so we had a shrewd idea how the situation was likely to resolve itself.

Olga suggested that we should leave Czechoslovakia. This came as a shock, as in the past when we discussed the possibility of emigrating she was always against such a move. Making such a decision is always a traumatic one and was especially so in her case because she was an only child who loved her parents dearly. Those who sympathized with the West were frequently vilified and punished in the Communist Bloc. Most Czech soldiers who fought against Hitler alongside the American, British or French troops during the Second World War were arrested and incarcerated in Communist concentration camps. So I may have been regarded as suspect, having recently spent two years in London. Olga knew this, so she was torn between staying to support her parents and leaving to avoid harm to me. She took charge, driving over to her mother and father to help her reach a decision. She told me she would go to see her parents and decide after gauging their reaction. If they said, 'We are glad you're still here', we would stay; but if they said, 'For Christ's sake, what are you doing here?' we would leave. Their response was the latter, and our fate was decided.

The first step was to obtain exit visas. When I had lectured the June before in London I had lost my passport. This was regarded as a terrible crime back in Prague. One was immediately suspected of selling such documents to the CIA or to MI5. Fortunately a colleague in Prague's university hospital had a contact at the Czech Foreign Office, a woman who helped me to replace it. Bribery was commonplace, so I handed over an envelope with £100 with my application for a replacement passport. This was a considerable amount of money back then. So now, applying for an exit visa, I went to see the same woman again. Queuing, I found myself sitting next to a Dutch journalist, and we got chatting. He said he was leaving the city that afternoon. I felt I could trust him, so I asked him if once he was across the border he could phone one of my hospital consultant colleagues in London – either Mr David Waterston or Mr Iain Aberdeen. I needed an invitation from one of them to come to London, which I would have to present to the authorities. The journalist did so, as promised – and I was to keep in touch with him for many years. At that time one of my friends from our department was spending six months at Great Ormond Street Hospital in central London. He helped the two consultants write an appropriate cable, as they had no idea how the

11

system in the Communist countries worked. They duly invited me to lecture at Great Ormond Street between 30 August and 7 September that year. I placed £200 in an envelope for my application for my exit visa, aware that I might get it but with an equal chance of being arrested. Fortunately I was successful, and three days later I was able to collect my documents.

Next I applied for an Austrian visa. The German border had been closed after the invasion, but the one adjoining Austria remained open for around three weeks. The surgery where Olga worked was opposite the Austrian Embassy. When I arrived there I found a queue of around 150 people. A few minutes later, when she looked out of the window again, there was no one to be seen. Her first thought was that we had all been arrested. Fortunately the Austrians had realized that we might be picked up and invited everyone into the inner court where we could not be seen from the street.

The Hippocratic Oath is integral to doctors' medical training, and helping patients to recover from their ailments is our priority. Two days after I applied for our Austrian visas I was presented with a patient with an inoperable kidney tumour. He needed a clot removed that was impeding the blood supply to his leg. I had no alternative but to take the patient to theatre. Just then I heard that our visas were ready for collection. I opened the groin, flushed the occluded artery and sutured it. But when I removed the clamps there was no pulse. So I repeated the procedure with the same result. The faster option was to ligate the artery, which might have resulted in a somewhat shorter leg. But as the boy had only a few months to live would that matter? I wanted to do the best for the child, so I persevered. The third time it worked. I rushed to collect the visas.

We packed swiftly that Friday. As the pretext for our journey was a week's lecturing in London we decided to take just one small suitcase so as not to raise suspicions. Our son was furious with his mother because she would not help him with his school homework for the following Monday, and he could not understand why. I went downstairs to the phone kiosk to call the Ministry of the Interior – at that time the most feared institution in the country. I asked if the border with Austria was still open, as we were supposed to drive to Vienna and then fly from there to London.

'Yes, sir, it is, but, as you probably know, things are not entirely in our hands. We don't know how long it will stay open. If you are planning to travel that way we would suggest you hurry.' This response was interesting. It

PROLOGUE: PRAGUE, 1968

revealed how the citizens of Prague, including members of the secret service educated in the USSR, were so upset by the invasion of Czechoslovakia they were prepared to assist those trying to leave the country.

We were anxious to make a safe escape. Would there be tanks in the woods near the border? We drove at top speed, as we did not know how long the border would remain open. Our hearts were in our mouths waiting for the inspection of our passports and visas. A few minutes' wait felt like an eternity.

But soon we were in Austria and were celebrating our escape with fellow émigrés and hugging strangers. At this point we informed Jaroslav that we were not going to London for a week but probably for much longer, to which he replied, 'Daddy, you're an amazing liar. I didn't realize a thing!' But when we told him that we were not flying but going by car he was less impressed. He had already driven with his mother from Prague to London when they had visited me the previous year and was plainly looking forward to travelling by air. Next he asked if he could go to school in Britain. Evidently his memories of the few weeks he had experienced at a London school had been good ones.

From Vienna I telephoned the hospital in Prague to inform my work associates that I had left and would no longer be on call. They took this news in their stride.

We found a cheap pension and got to work arranging German and Belgian transit visas and entry visas to Britain. With the help of friends we managed to buy ferry tickets from Ostend to Dover. With these our transit visas were a mere formality, and British visas was swiftly granted. I had worked in the London for two years, and my consultants there had informed the authorities and made assurances for me. We drove through Germany and stopped in Bonn, where I called Carlo Kallfelz, a paediatric cardiologist who had spent several months in the cardiac department in London. He sounded very emotional at the end of the phone but instructed us to drive to the main square where he would collect us. Indeed he was so excited and nervous that he turned up in his slippers.

Carlo and his wife Imgaard were tremendously warm and welcoming. After two days of recovering with them we continued on our journey. They packed our car with blankets, cutlery and pillows – just about everything that you could think of that would fit into our little Fiat – and off we went. Largely thanks to them the final lap of our journey to London went without hitch.

13

1
CHILDHOOD
1934–1945

I was born in Prague in 1934. I was premature with a large cephalohaematoma on my skull. Apparently my paternal grandmother visited the family shortly after I arrived. She took one look at me and told my mother, 'Jiřina, you must be philosophical. Think of it like this. You have a beautiful vase. It is broken, so you get another one.' My mother never forgave her.

My father was a very successful dental surgeon, and my mother worked as his assistant, but after my younger sister was born she gave up work to look after both of us. My paternal grandfather was an official at the Finance Ministry, while his wife was a concert pianist. So from an early age I took piano lessons with her, but as I did not have a musical ear I detested these. Fortunately my grandmother was a keen chess player, and I discovered that if I turned up with an interesting chess problem this shortened the lesson considerably. My father had two sisters. Mařička was a paediatrician, but Lojzička had had brain damage from birth. She lived with my grandparents and occasionally became violent. My grandmother treated her more like a servant or a second-class citizen than as a daughter. In her later years, after my grandparents had died, she was sent to a psychiatric establishment, where the family visited her once a week. It was very sad.

My mother's father was a decorator, a lovely man who smoked like a chimney and died of a coronary attack at a relatively young age. My maternal grandmother was a saint. She was a fantastic cook and an extremely kind person who would help my mother with everything. It was only as I grew up that I realized she had been exploited by my parents, who took advantage of her good nature. My mother had a brother, Franta, who lived outside Prague, but we did not see much of him. She also had a younger sister Eva, who studied chemistry at Charles University in Prague. She completed her first year, but then the Germans occupied the country and closed the universities. At this point she started helping my grandfather in his business. After the war she felt that she was too old to recommence her studies, which

I thought was a mistake. Her parents interfered with her choice of boyfriends, so one day she decided to show them that she could make up her own mind. She was at the time dating a man twenty years her senior, and out of the blue she married him. I think they had a reasonable marriage, but I felt she deserved better. They had two boys, Honza and Tomáš, but we did not meet them often.

My father's courtship of my mother was somewhat bizarre. After about four years of dating he told her they should stop seeing one another. He said he was going to look around to see if he could find someone better than her; if not, he would come back. Anyway after around two years he returned, and my mother took him back and accepted his proposal of marriage. When I was told about this at first I was incredulous, but then I thought it was typical of my father, as he always put himself first. Another instance of this manifested some years later when he bought my mother a birthday present of four spare tyres for his car.

In 1939 he built a summer-house in Senohraby, a popular village for people from Prague to spend their summers. He draw out rough plans for a Spanish-style hacienda and presented them to an architect friend who rejected them as unworkable but came back two weeks later saying that on second thoughts they were probably fine. So the villa was built to my father's specifications. My earliest recollections of the construction is how my sister who was four and I, aged seven, would help cement stones on the patio in front of the villa and plant shrubs and trees. Today the trees are around 20 metres high. The village is about 30 kilometres from Prague and well connected by rail. During the war we were not allowed to drive cars, so trains were the only available means of transport. Later on the Germans were even to confiscate people's skis for their winter troops.

My first encounter with religion was during my first year at primary school in Prague after the Germans occupied the country. We had to learn their language. Soon after subjects such as history and geography were taught in German. After the first year we all had to go to confession. My parents were Roman Catholics but, as I later remarked, 'Catholics just in case there was something in it'. We children did not understand the concept of sin. I remember sitting outside the church with my schoolmates; we had been told to list our sins, and we were copying them from one another. After I finished my first year my mother, sister and I moved permanently to

Senohraby, where I finished my primary education. We expected Prague to be bombed, and my father felt it would be safer for us in the country.

One of my first memories from that time was my parents' so-called 'divorce'. Couples were not allowed to have two houses or apartments, so my parents' solution was to get divorced. My father lived and worked in Prague; my mother lived with us in Senohraby. This was the first time that my sister and I had conflicts about telling the truth. My father had official visiting rights one weekend a month, but he came every Friday evening and did not leave until Monday morning. We had been told always to be truthful, but we could not say that our father was with us each weekend. Meanwhile all radios were modified to disable the short wave so that we could not listen to the BBC or Voice of America. But people worked out how to have short wave reinstalled by friendly engineers. Being caught listening to foreign broadcasts carried a penalty of imprisonment and potential deportation to a concentration camp. We had to learn quickly which type of truth was for domestic use and which was for the outside world.

At the beginning of the war my father was trying to think of a disease to claim that he had that could not easily be detected but which would prevent him from being drafted to work in Germany. He decided on neuralgia of the trigeminus or fifth cranial nerve, which causes severe attacks of pain. We could not believe it when around three weeks later he actually started suffering from the condition. The pain must have been unbearable, as he had to lock himself in a spare room where we could not hear his screams. He subsequently underwent an operation that involved electrocoagulation of the Gasserian ganglion at the base of the brain. It was a stereotaxic operation during which they guide a needle through a little foramen at the base of the skull into the ganglion and then pass an electric current through it. He had this procedure done twice but with only temporary relief. After the war he decided to have an open operation, which was conducted in Hradec Králové by Professor Petr, a well-known neurosurgeon, and this was successful.

I experienced a further conflict with religion in Senohraby when a very strict priest who gave us religious instruction at school expected us to attend mass each Sunday. The church was in a neighbouring village about 5 kilometres away, so my father urged me not to go, saying that he was only around for the weekend and that God would forgive me. But I was petrified each Monday when the priest would ask whether we had attended mass. I think it was the beginning of my drift away from the church.

School was great fun. We had two classrooms: in the first, years one, two and three were taught; in the second, years four and five had their lessons. When one year was reading, the other was writing and the third did homework. Our breaks were spent either kicking footballs on the street outside or playing cops and robbers in the school's large garden. On our way home we would sometimes dawdle for two or three hours instead of returning within fifteen minutes. No one seemed to mind. We would catch lizards and scrump apples or cherries, depending on the season. In winter I would go to school on skis, as there was usually quite a lot of snow.

In the summer we spent the afternoons at the Sázava River, a fifteen-minute walk from our house. There was a pleasant swimming club that had changing cabins. Each family had its own, as there was no communal changing facility. Table tennis was a favourite activity, and we kept a canoe there. We fished for trout, and as we did not have a licence one of us would have to be on the look-out for the authorities. My younger sister would sometimes accompany us. I remember one Sunday morning we were fishing in a brook near the river where there was a good deep pool in which we often managed to catch a trout or two. My sister, by then five or six, fell into the brook, so that was the end of the fishing for the day; we made a swift retreat to dry her off.

Next to our garden was our neighbours' garden belonging to Jiřina Šejbalová, a famous actress in the Czech National Theatre, and her husband Jarda Pipek. They had a volleyball court where we played volleyball as well as noheyball, which was football across a low net. We very much enjoyed these activities.

In 1944 I sat the entrance examinations to grammar school. First, I had to sit an entry examination to the secondary modern, and only after passing that was I allowed to sit a second one for the grammar school. The headmaster in our village school had suggested to my parents that I should not even bother to sit the examination. Since the primary school had just two classrooms he felt the standard of teaching would not be as good as elsewhere. But my parents and I thought that there was nothing to lose by trying. To his great surprise I passed. The school was in Prague – in Nerudova Street in Malá Strana (Lesser Town) – so I used to travel by train to Prague with my father. At lunchtime I would prepare lunch for him, as he worked at the surgery the whole day. One of his favourite dishes was cauliflower eggs – a dish I could not bring myself to consume for many years afterwards. During one of our train trips to Prague my father carried a flat box with flour and butter on his chest and another one with eggs and other provisions on his back purchased illicitly from a friendly farmer who lived near our village. My father had the two boxes covered by his old leather greatcoat. But walking through a foot tunnel in Prague's main station was nerve-racking. On both sides of the exit we would see SS soldiers on guard duty. I knew that if my father were caught with the contraband food it would mean deportation to a concentration camp – a terrifying thought for a ten-year-old.

The school authorities decided after a few months that because of the chance of air raids it was too dangerous for us to attend school every day. On Fridays we would go in to collect our homework for the week, and the following Friday we would bring it back. As I was living now in Senohraby that suited me well. My friend Jindra Beránek would bring all the papers to my father, who came back to us every Friday. I would do the homework over the weekend, and Jindra would collect it from my father and take it in the following Friday. It was quite a leisurely existence.

In the spring of 1945 we watched the Allied bombers flying over to bomb the German cities. We loved to collect the silver-foil strips the Allied planes dropped to fool the German radar. Later on I would go down to the railway tracks with my sister to watch the passing trains. The railway was a short run across the meadow and through a small wood. My sister, aged eight, and I, eleven, watched the German trains transporting prisoners from the eastern concentration camps to the west. It was horrific. The cattle wagons were sealed, but in places one could see an arm or a leg dressed in concentration-camp uniform sticking out. We were not sure whether the occupants of the wagons were alive or dead.

Then came the Prague Uprising on 5 May. My father went to work as a doctor at the local partisan unit. We followed developments with our mother via the radio. There were a few tense moments. When the Prague radio called for help with medical supplies my father's unit captured a large depot of medicines near by. He took the supplies and drove in an ambulance to a hospital in Prague. On the way they encountered several German units and

Vlasov's units – Russian units fighting alongside the Germans under General Vlasov. Both the Vlasov units and the Germans were determined to confiscate the medical supplies, so it was a miracle that my father was able to deliver them to the Krč Hospital in Prague. On 6 or 7 May Prague radio asked for urgent help. The US's General Patton was about 50 kilometres west of Prague, and in no time he reached its outskirts to liberate the city. Unfortunately at this point he received orders to go back to Plzeň (Pilsen), which was on the line agreed at the Yalta Conference between Stalin and the Allies. At that time the Soviet army under General Zhukov was about 200 kilometres east of Prague, and it took him another two days to reach the city. During this time the waste of human life was unbelievable, and the destruction of buildings wrought by the Germans was devastating.

Shortly after VE Day part of our villa in Senohraby was requisitioned for use by the Russian army as a command post. At first, the Russians were friendly. They placed a large barrel with methylated spirit under the rockery, and most of the time a Russian soldier lay under this with one end of a piece of rubber tube in his mouth, while the other end was connected to the barrel.

After about a month the Russians left. They gave my friend Jirka Vorlíček and myself a horse each. These were rather elderly ones, but they became useful when Jirka's family returned home. They had had to leave their farm during the war, as the area had been used as a German artillery shooting range.

I will never forget the night the Russians left. They stole the keys from all the rooms, cut out and removed the leather from our settees in the reception room. They also cut their initials with their bayonets into our beautiful dining table.

Things then really escalated. They attempted to rape my mother. Fortunately my father had left one of his service revolvers with her, and she managed to protect herself and see them off without harm.

2
POST-WAR YEARS, 1945–1947

The first few years after the war were exciting ones for me. There was rationing, but we were free. We lived in Pařížská Street, the main road leading from the Old Town Square to the river. Before the war it was called Mikulášká Street, later renamed Pařížská. The Germans changed most street names, so ours became Norimberska, to revert once more to Pařížská at the end of wartime. Thankfully the Russians did not change the name again when they invaded in 1968.

When I was eleven I started attending Dušní Grammar School, in the same block as our apartment – it took all of two minutes to get there.

In June 1945 my friend Jindra Beránek and I looked for a Boy Scouts unit to join. We found Středisko Šipka, which had its centre on Senovážne Námestí. The two of us enrolled in a cub unit, and in August we departed for our first summer camp. We slept on straw mattresses in the local school. One of our activities involved helping local farmers with the harvest, but we were also initiated into the scouting life and ethos, with all its tests, night marches, first aid and so on. We found it highly enjoyable and absorbing.

I will never forget the day when during the morning roll call we were informed that Japan had capitulated and that war was over. I also remember vividly when we started receiving assistance from United Nations Relief And Rehabilitation Administration, known as UNRRA. This included a variety of foodstuffs with which the Americans were trying to aid the malnourished or starving people of post-war Europe. For me the best items to arrive were small tins of canned peaches and peanut butter, neither of which we had tasted before.

The next year, 1946, while we were cub scouts we attended a summer camp at little Lake Člunek in southern Bohemia. We slept in the loft of a barn, while the senior scouts had their tents near by. We enjoyed camp life greatly. In the woods we discovered juicy blackberries and wonderful *hříbky*, or cep, mushrooms that we collected to supplement our meals. During the autumn we were involved in raising money to rebuild the clubhouse. We acquired an old building in Petřín Park, a stone's throw from the US embassy, and as our main source of income we collected and sold wine bottles. I recall the discovery of the cellar of my parents' friends, Dr Pipek and his wife, the actress Jiřina Šejbalová. They lived two houses away from us in Pařížská Street. They were heavy drinkers, and we amassed more than 200 wine bottles from their cellar. Another source of income was the selling of cards that were designed to look like bricks (*cihly* in Czech). Our scouting activities occupied us fully, including outings every weekend to the suburbs of Prague. In the summer of 1947 my parents went on holiday to Yugoslavia, but I refused to accompany them, as I preferred to go to the scouts' summer camp in Holná, another lake in southern Bohemia.

Our original group leader was Ruda, an old friend of mine with whom we had gone winter skiing for a few years. By the time of the summer camp in Holná I had been promoted to scout group leader, while Ruda had been appointed deputy leader of the whole outfit.

Every third day I was in charge of meals for about forty hungry youngsters. It was a major task to feed them all, but we managed to satisfy everyone. A good test was a day when we had to prepare around 200 blueberry dumplings. Fortunately everyone liked them.

Most of us knew one another already, as we had been cubs together and had attended the same school. During the summer camp I took the test known as 'Three Eagle Feathers', which consisted of a day of not talking and not eating, a day hiding somewhere and not being spotted by anyone and a night of sleeping rough in the woods. Not talking was a particular challenge, as the other boys would continually encourage the individual being tested to say something or to respond to casual queries. But I passed.

At the end of the summer camp we took a trip in our little boats, called *pramičky*, on the Vltava river back to Prague. The boats could take five, at a push, seven boys – six rowers and one person steering. We were negotiating a lock one time with a boy called Standa Galíček, who was an extra body on board. He was sitting at the front of the vessel on top of our baggage, and around his neck was a plastic folder containing our food coupons. When he thought the boat was going to capsize he took a mighty jump from the vessel to the edge of the lock some distance away. Belatedly he realized that we might lose our precious coupons. We did indeed overturn the boat – but he succeeded in saving the coupons, so all was forgiven.

3
COMMUNIST TAKEOVER, 1948

February 1948 was a period when everything changed. There was a highly active Communist Party in Czechoslovakia, and during the 1947 elections the party emerged as dominant, although it did not have a majority. This was undoubtedly a consequence of the Munich Agreement or Treaty of 1938. Many intellectuals and the middle classes were disillusioned by what they regarded as the 'betrayal' by England and France at this time. We had a pact of mutual assistance, and, although we knew that these countries were no match for Hitler, selling us down the river was long remembered, in particular Chamberlain's description of Czechoslovakia as 'a far-away country of which we British know little'. Many at this point transferred their allegiance to the USSR. There was a feeling that as a small nation we needed a powerful ally. But of course it was the wrong choice; the atrocities Stalin had perpetrated on his own people were already widely known.

During the elections of 1948 the Communist Party received a substantial vote, and in February they staged a *putsch*. Several right and centre ministers offered their resignation, which was accepted by President Beneš. The Communist leader Gottwald thus became president. And from then on things started going downhill rapidly.

Soon after the Communist takeover I was interrogated for six hours at the secret-police headquarters in Bartolomějská Street. The Boy Scouts organization was considered bourgeois, and the fact that its founder, Robert Baden-Powell, had first established it in Britain did not help. As a group leader I was regarded as suspect, and dozens of questions had to be answered. It was not a pleasant experience for a fourteen-year-old.

At school the curriculum was rewritten. It was no longer Edison who invented the electric light bulb; it was Ševčenko. It was not Stevenson who invented the steam engine; it was Kravčenko. We were not allowed to learn about Mendel, nor about genetics, only about Lysenko and Pavlov. At school Russian became the second language. At the beginning of each lesson the teachers had to put up a quote from Marx, Engels, Lenin or Stalin on the blackboard. That included physical education classes. No one was safe. There was at least one informer in each class. His or her report could ruin your education and career prospects.

During the summer holidays, as the Brigade of Socialist Work, we had to undertake manual work, picking hops, working in the factories and so on. Harvesting hops was an unpleasant business. Hops are sticky, and pulling the plants down creates a cloud of dust. But generally the work was not too bad, as we enjoyed the companionship and had some fun. Also we were at an age when chasing the opposite sex was on the agenda, and as our classes were co-educational girls attended the summer camps as well.

One year my friends from the scout group and I decided to organize the summer work ourselves. In order to avoid problems with officialdom we asked a boy from the fifth form, a Communist, to join us. He was a rather jolly lad, not intent on pushing his politics too much. We travelled to Harrachov in the Krkonoše Mountains where we were to prepare the terrain for the construction of a major new road.

Our Communist associate was interested in zoology, particularly in snakes, and he taught us how to catch vipers without being bitten. Things went wrong when he decided that in order to develop immunity he needed to let one bite him. He had between six and eight snakes in a bag under his bed. One evening at around 7.30 he released one, let it bite a cloth and then bite him. I was leader of the group and felt responsible, so I summoned the local doctor. When he arrived he gave my friend some antidote serum and asked how he had got bitten. The lad was at first evasive but eventually said that if the doctor promised not to make a fuss he would tell him. After receiving assurances that he would not get in trouble he took the bag from under his bed and produced the captive vipers. You should have seen the doctor's face. A month later our friend gave us each a viper, which we brought home in a jam jar. You cannot imagine the reaction of my mother when three days later mine produced six babies. The next day, under strict orders, I took them to Prague Zoo.

Not everything was grim during those Communist years. We had fun, especially when it came to sport. We had our local sports days, or *spartakiads*, where we participated in a number of activities. First, one ran 60 metres, followed by a long jump before one was called on to participate in a volleyball or basketball match or whatever. I was a keen skier, both downhill and slalom, as my father had started teaching me when I was two and a half years old. Generally we looked on those who favoured cross-country skiing as inferior, because they had to slog so hard to get anywhere. Of course this sometimes applied to us. There were very few ski lifts, so often during competitions we had to climb mountains with the skis on our back. As a result we could usually manage no more than two training runs a day.

Around the time I was sixteen my father gave me cross-country skis for Christmas and entered me into the county cross-country championships the following February. With my competitive spirit I trained hard and succeeded in winning the county championships in my age category. By the time I was seventeen I thought I had a good chance of doing well in the national downhill and slalom championships. I attended the county championships in Harrachov. It was a difficult run, particularly at a right-hand bend that sloped to the left. I often fell there, but as there was considerable fresh snow it was like falling into a duvet. Unfortunately in my youthful enthusiasm – or should I say stupidity? – I decided to undertake a run late in the afternoon before the race the following day. I went full tilt and fell at the bend, but because by now the piste had been prepared for the race the snow was hard and impacted, and when I fell I skidded straight into the woods. Not only did I break my leg at the fibula but I ruined my skis, and they were very expensive and not easy to obtain. I was transported down the mountain on a small sledge with my broken leg strapped to it, which was a gruelling experience as I was in agony all the way.

My friend from the ski club won the race the next day, while I was put in plaster. Three weeks later he won the downhill at the national championship in our age category. I was in plaster for four weeks, then had to undergo physiotherapy for ten days. After this I entered our club's slalom competition. To my great delight I somehow managed to beat my friend, the champion, by almost two seconds.

My sister Jiřina was three years younger than me and another very good skier, and we had wonderful times skiing as a family. My parents were excellent skiers and taught us the basic techniques, and we got to know well the ski slopes in Krkonoše or Giant Mountains and in the Low Tatra mountains in Slovakia.

When Jiřina finished school she trained as a physiotherapist. We had not been especially close as children, but, after a separation of twenty-one years, by which time I was well established as a cardiac surgeon in London, we bonded immediately, and after our reunion our relationship went from strength to strength.

I played tennis, volleyball and basketball, but my preferred sport remained skiing. During the seventh and eighth form at school I was heavily involved in training. In summer we had a session each week in the Tirš house on Malá Strana. It was the training of the junior national team that was especially hard as it consisted of interval training, which was introduced into the sport by Emil Zátopek, a famous long-distance runner. He had won the 5,000 and 10,000 metres and the marathon at the Helsinki Olympics. Moreover his wife Dana had won the gold medal in the javelin event, so they were a well-known couple.

Our training consisted of several 60-metre runs, each interrupted by a minute's rest, then exercises to strengthen the upper body, then running 400 metres a few times and back for press-ups. As I liked to stay fit I cycled to and from the training from Senohraby some 30 kilometres from Prague.

When winter arrived we had ski camp for ten days before Christmas, then we went off with our parents over the holidays. Our family usually celebrated Christmas Eve a week early so that we could have ten days of uninterrupted skiing. Subsequently there was a competition one week, then training a week or two later and on and on. It was extremely enjoyable, but once I enrolled in medical school I could not spend three months skiing as it was not compatible with my studies.

One Easter I went skiing to Krkonoše with my father and his friends. We had lunch in Klinovky, an area with mountain huts that included a restaurant. My father ordered a steak. It was very tough, so he summoned the waiter. 'D'you have a tiger here?' my father asked. The man was perplexed. My father continued, 'Only a tiger could chew your steaks!'

It was always tricky to return to school from skiing with a sick note and a suntan. On one occasion I did not know what excuse my father had made for my absence. When the teacher muttered a Latin word I couldn't catch, looked at me and said, 'Well, your father's a medic so he knows what he has written', I had an anxious few seconds. I might have said I had a sore throat, but my father had written 'diarrhoea'.

I continued going on river trips for several years with our scout group and also set up a private poetry and discussion group. But such activity had to be kept strictly secret, as its discovery would have resulted in expulsion from school – if not a far worse punishment.

While I was in the sixth form I started dating Dana, a congenial girl a year my junior who lived two houses away in the same street. She was very good at sport, especially gymnastics, and we used to play tennis and go running together to Letná Park and Malá Strana in our tracksuits. We saw each other four or five times a week, but her mother was very strict, so she had to get home early. A popular place to take your girlfriend at that time was the opera, which was regarded as the 'in thing'. Everyone would wear their best clothes to attend, although I did not own a suit, and we usually stood in the gods.

In summer three or four of us had enjoyable holidays hitchhiking to Slovakia to the High and Low Tatras. There were usually a few of us with or without girlfriends. We would hitch rides by placing the most attractive girl by the side of the road while the rest of us would duck down in a nearby ditch. When a lorry stopped the driver would be surprised when we all jumped out and climbed aboard. We lived and camped very simply; our tents didn't even have groundsheets.

Our final year at the grammar school came in 1952, by which time I was eighteen. Matriculation was the equivalent of A levels in the UK but included more subjects. We all had to study the Czech and Russian languages and mathematics. Then there was a choice, and I opted for geography, French and biology, in which I did well.

After getting my results I applied for medical school without much hope. With my background, my father being a dental surgeon and therefore regarded as bourgeois, I thought my chances of acceptance were slim. So, as a second choice, I put down the Military Medical Academy – even though I hated anything militaristic – as I felt my chances of being accepted to study medicine there was better.

Included in the application to the university was a character reference from the local Communist Party member. That person in our block of flats was the wife of the concierge and stoker. She cleaned our apartment regularly for years, so she was a family friend. She was an uneducated but very kind woman, and when she was asked to provide a reference she came to see me with the forms she had received. She handed them to me and said, 'Jarouŝku [a diminutive of Jaroslav], I have no clue how to write this. Why don't you write it yourself?' I was lucky, but I knew several friends where such references had destroyed their career prospects. My first wife Olga later told me that in her class in Pardubice there had been a Communist activist who had provided awful, damning references for all her fellow students. When the headmistress read them she decided that they should be revised. She took it upon herself to rewrite them all. With the original references, probably no one would have got to university. The headmistress was a pre-war Communist with high ideals and common sense, so her pupils were fortunate.

I was in Senohraby, enjoying the summer but apprehensive about my chances of studying medicine. Finally one July morning the postman came to my father's villa with a registered letter. I had been accepted by Charles University Medical School.

4
MEDICAL SCHOOL, 1952–1958

We started our studies in September 1952. We were divided into study groups of twenty to twenty-five students, and each group had a student leader and a political leader. The political leaders were recruited mainly from the ADK (Absolvent Dělnických Kursů); they were graduates of workers' courses organized by the Communist Party. Youngsters with no previous education were rushed through a one-year course, at the end of which they passed their matriculation examinations. Then the party ordered them to study medicine, law, engineering or whatever at the university, irrespective of whether they had any interest in or aptitude for that particular subject. We were fortunate that our political leader was a decent person, mild-mannered and grateful for any help we could offer him with his studies. He was clearly not up to the medical course, but he tried hard. When the time came for him to write up individual political profiles and assessments, like the wife of the concierge and stoker at our block of flats he came to me and said, 'Jarda, I haven't a clue how to write this. Why don't you do it yourself?' After the first two years he switched to dentistry and eventually became my parents-in-law's dentist. In this profession he was good, caring and very popular.

Our curriculum reflected the political system. The first two years we had to study the Russian language and political economy. We had two hours a week in each of those subjects and no longer than that on anatomy and pathology. We had to register our names as confirmation of our presence at lectures and seminars, so for the lectures in Marxist philosophy one of us would sign in for the other four. I will never forget when after about nine months Honza Stupka, a member of our group, was surprised to learn that the second name of a fellow student, Olga, was Slugová. He had been signing her in as Sluková!

After I was dumped by my girlfriend Dana I was devastated. However, during my second year at medical school I started going out with Olga. She was from Pardubice, where her father was a schoolteacher. Her mother, also trained as a teacher, worked as an administrator at a meat factory. (Pardubice was to become quite famous, initially for hosting one of the best steeplechase races in the country but later for having a factory that manufactured Semtex, an explosive used by terrorist groups round the world.) Olga was very keen on rowing. She was country champion in eights a few times and very good in a skiff. When we first met she was seeing a young man from her rowing club in her home town, but before long we started going out together.

I spent the first two years of my medical studies as a demonstrator at the Institute of Anatomy. I decided that anatomy was crucial if I was to specialize in surgery, which was my ambition. The first project assigned to me and to my colleague Zdena Synkova, a student from the same study group, was the dissection of penile veins!

Some of our professors were great characters. Professor Richter taught inorganic chemistry. He took us one day to Petřín Park and under the statue of Mácha he scribbled chemical formulas on the asphalt paths. This was pretty unusual behaviour, because it was a location better known as a May Day rendezvous for courting couples. He was a tough examiner, and it was a great achievement to pass one of his tests. Another memorable individual was Professor Hepner who taught pathological physiology. He came to the laboratory where we were working one day and asked questions on his subject – mostly trick questions. As I was a student leader I was the first in the line of fire, and I gave a wrong answer. He said to me, 'You have to think in a logical way. Memorizing is not good enough. If I asked you the branches of the profunda femoral artery you wouldn't have a clue.' Without hesitation I recited the names of the branches. He fell quiet. 'You are not by any chance a demonstrator at the Institute of Anatomy, are you?' When I confirmed that I was he was delighted that he had deduced this with his logical mind.

In order to avoid two years of military service, one morning a week we did military theory and attended a month's military summer camp after years two and four. This meant that after we finished medical school we would be called only for six months instead of two years, already having a few pips on our shoulders. We were then usually placed as military unit doctors. This meant that we had a modicum of independence. After the second year we had a month of military indoctrination in a camp near Jičín in northern Bohemia. The young officers hated the students and did everything to make our lives miserable, such as making us go on our stomachs through mud and pools of water, complaining about our poor bed-making technique and so on. But we knew that we only had to endure this for a month, so we took it on the chin and kept smiling.

I continued to go skiing around Christmas, at half-term and at Easter. These were great trips with my best friends. One year we went to Chopok in the Low Tatras; it was fantastic skiing terrain, as the mountains were generally covered by grass under the snow and not rocks as in the High Tatras. The highest mountain was 2,200 metres, perfect for skiing. We were staying in a little hut about twenty minutes' walk from the lifts with twelve bunk beds in a single large room. There was a small stove in the middle, but at night it would get very cold. I remember one morning a girlfriend of my friend Vojta Volavka woke up with her hair frozen and stuck to the window. As we had to wash in a brook outside the hut life was tough. In the morning, if the temperature was lower than –20 degrees centigrade we would wait a while before walking to the chairlift, and when it was that cold the attendants would place a blanket over our shoulders.

My good friend Vojta was a very bright young man with great wit which in later years reminded me of the mordant humour of Woody Allen. He was the son of a professor of art history who wrote interesting books on Czech paintings of the nineteenth and twentieth centuries. His mother was a director of the Jewish Museum in Prague, a well-known and highly respected cultural institution. Later on, after he emigrated to the USA, when he mentioned that his name was Volavka all doors opened up to him.

At the end of the war Vojta was imprisoned with his father in the notorious Prison Na Pankráci, known as Pečkárna. Being half-Jewish, they were awaiting transport to a concentration camp and scheduled to leave Prague on 6 May. While incarcerated at the prison his father taught him Hebrew and Jewish history. Fortunately for them the Prague Uprising began on 5 May, so they never made it on to the transport train.

One day in his second year a meeting of medical students with the dean of the Medical School, Professor Trávníček, took place. During the debate Vojta asked some pointed questions and made a fool of the dean. By the time Vojta walked out of the room he was convinced he would be expelled from medical school. The following day he was due to sit a very tricky examination in pathology. He went on a drinking spree the previous night and wandered aimlessly around Prague thinking all was lost. In the morning he was woken up by a phone call from a fellow student asking why he wasn't at the examination. Vojta replied that it was pointless as he was going to be thrown out. His friend informed him that some teachers had spoken to the dean and persuaded him to reconsider. Vojta was not to be expelled, and the examiner was waiting for him at the Institute of Pathology. Vojta rushed in, still somewhat the worse for wear for drink, but to his surprise he passed the examination. In fact we students suspected that Doc Žahoř had probably ensured that he got through, as he had admired his stance against the dean.

Vojta's cousin was a researcher at the Jewish Museum in Prague. One evening she was walking from the museum through a narrow dark street in the Old Town. She heard whispering behind her and realized that a man was running to catch up with her. She was frightened, so she took flight, but he caught up with her. Very politely he asked, 'Excuse me, miss, are you by any chance a prostitute?' Appalled, she continued walking but overheard him running back and saying to his male companion, 'You idiot. I told you whores don't wear spectacles!'

5
GRADUATION AND FIRST YEAR OF MEDICAL PRACTICE, 1958

Olga and I graduated in 1958. I was twenty-four. I gained top marks in all three subjects: medicine, surgery, and obstetrics and gynaecology. Afterwards all the jobs available to us were posted at the deanery. I decided to apply for a surgical position in Benešov, which had a good district general hospital where I had practised two summers previously as a medical student. A young surgeon, Pavel Scheck, assisted me with my first appendectomy there. He subsequently emigrated to Holland where he became a successful anaesthetist in Rotterdam and where his wife Hanka was a cardiologist. One time they came to England to visit, and we played golf together. It was very good to see him again.

In the hospital at Benešov there were four posts for house surgeons available and five candidates. As I was the only person whom the head of the department knew and supported, and the only one to graduate with honours, I was reasonably confident of getting the position. Olga, meanwhile, had applied for a post in paediatric neurology in a hospital less than half an hour away. But I was the only one of the five candidates who did not get a job. Neither did Olga get hers. Our political views and our middle-class backgrounds seemed to be the major stumbling block. We learned later that the reason we did not get the positions was that one of Olga's colleagues had given us a poor character reference purely out of spite.

In the second round I applied for a post in the north of the country, Nová Paka. Professor Bohuslav Niederle, the best general surgeon in Prague and a schoolmate of my father, had recommended it to me as a good hospital. I knew Professor Niederle from his visits to my parents at home, and when I was in the fifth year of medical school he had handed me a rough draft of his new book *Acute Abdomen* for my comments. I had been practising regularly in several surgical departments during the previous three years and

GRADUATION AND FIRST YEAR OF MEDICAL PRACTICE, 1958

read around the subject a great deal, so I took the task very seriously. I made a number of suggestions where I felt things were unclear or where there might be errors, and the professor was impressed. He thanked me profusely in the foreword, as others he had asked to read the book had merely responded with generalized compliments and platitudes.

Olga eventually got a position in Košumberk, a sanatorium specializing in tuberculosis of the bones in children. Our good friend Franta Piťha got a job there as well, so at least she had companionship. It was in the eastern part of the country not far from my hospital, but train connections were poor. It used to take about four hours to visit one another, even though the distance was barely 120 kilometres.

My job proved a disaster. I had been interested in surgery for a number of years and had been practising in surgical departments in Prague (Na Františku), the Department of Surgery in Benešov and the Clinic of Paediatric Surgery (Na Karlově) where paediatric cardiac surgery was also carried out. But the head, my boss in Nová Paka, had achieved his high position at a very young age because he had married the former boss's daughter. On the day I arrived, his secretary at the urology out-patients, where the boss was working, sent me in. He pointed at a metal rotating stool and said, 'Do sit down, Charlie.' He called all his juniors 'Charlie'. After about ten minutes he said, 'You can get up. The stool should be warm by now!' And things didn't improve after that. When I was working in A&E a patient came in with an advanced infection under the thumbnail. I made an incision, removed the pus and prescribed penicillin. Before my shift was finished my boss summoned me to his office and reprimanded me for wasting public money. Instead of the 300,000 units I had prescribed, he said that 30,000 units would have been sufficient.

Once when he had been away we saw a patient who developed septicaemia after a prostatic resection. My senior colleague, Dr Mihula, did a cystoscopy, catheterized the ureter and took a sample of pus from the renal pelvis. While we were taking the sample to the ambulance for transport to the laboratory in the university hospital in Hradec Králové we encountered our boss who asked what we were carrying. When we explained, he snatched the sample and threw it away, shouting, 'What on earth would they think of us at the teaching hospital?' His attitude was disgraceful. One time I was on call when a 21-year-old man presented with acute appendicitis. I clerked him in and called the boss. I described the patient's vital signs – all classic signs of appendicitis – and expected that he would ask me to set up the operating-room in readiness for surgery. Instead he commanded, 'Charlie, place the patient under a sheet soaked with vinegar and cold water and call me in two hours.' As instructed I phoned him at that time. By then the patient's pulse was racing and his temperature soaring. But it was another three hours before my boss arrived to perform the appendectomy.

6
MILITARY SERVICE, 1958–1959

Fortunately I did not stay in the post at Nová Paka for long. Three months later I was called for my six months' military service. I had been assigned to a unit near Dětřichov, in Orlické hory in the Moravian mountains, to replace a doctor who had spent a full two years there.

The unit was basically divided in two. The majority of personnel there were infantry, their main task being to guard the large ammunition depot. We were told that if the depot exploded all the windows in the town of Olomouc would go. And Olomouc was around 40 kilometres away. The second group was a small detachment of airmen whose commander was a major and therefore commander of the entire outfit.

I was attached to the infantry, and my commander was a captain. As I was the first doctor to be seconded to the unit for just six months no one had much idea of my main duties. So it was not too difficult to persuade my commander that I was entitled to spend a day a week in the local hospital as part of my professional development. Soon after I started he asked me if I would participate in the officers' weekend duty rota. They wanted to return home to see their families, while I was stuck there anyway. I was only a sergeant, but being a doctor carried the status of captain, so I agreed because I thought it might be a useful bargaining tool. Moreover I used to play ice hockey for a top junior team in Prague, and my commander was a keen ice hockey player and fan. He entered our team into a local military unit competition, and I recall his excitement when I scored my first goal.

One day the captain called me and said they expected a visit from divisional headquarters, so I could not take my scheduled leave the following weekend. I was furious, as Olga had arranged to have the same weekend off, and we had hoped to meet in Prague. Fortunately I recalled what my

37

predecessor had advised before he left, so I sat down in my office in the sick bay and wrote a note to the captain saying that I had inspected the latrines and regarded them as an epidemic risk. I said that they should be dug up and replaced within twenty-four hours. Half an hour later I was summoned to see him. He screamed and ranted, but after a few minutes he scrutinized me thoughtfully and asked, 'Does this have anything to do with your cancelled leave?' 'Well . . . maybe,' I replied, eventually. At that he handed me back my note and said, 'Tear it up and take your leave. OK?'

Once a week I undertook surgery in a nearby village. My predecessor had done so, and as there was no doctor there it was much appreciated by the population. This also gave me considerable freedom. I would visit remote farms to see sick patients on cross-country skis, as it was winter. Out in the heart of the countryside a farmer would regularly slaughter a pig. So while I was attending my patients I could participate in a feast of roast pig, black pudding and other porcine titbits (in Czech, *zabíjačka*) – washed down with plentiful local drink.

One day the commanding major of the air force summoned me to his office and told me that as I was meant to be undertaking basic military training it was unacceptable that I was going in and out of the military area as I pleased. So no more 'doctoring' in the village. When I told him my predecessor had been holding regular surgeries there for a number of years he was uninterested. 'That's their problem' was his reply.

He left that afternoon for a divisional meeting. Early the same evening his wife phoned me. Officers' families lived in a newly constructed block of flats on the outskirts of the village, and she asked me if I could come over and examine her five-year-old son who was running a very high temperature. I explained that her husband had prohibited me from leaving the military zone. She was furious and desperate. As she pleaded with me to come anyway I said I would but that I hoped I would not be court-martialled.

The boy had tonsillitis, so aspirin and a shot of penicillin sorted things out. The day after the major returned I was summoned to his office. With a stern face he thanked me for what I had done for his son and informed me that from the following week I could resume my surgery in the village.

Around this time I entered an army skiing contest in the beautiful Beskydy mountain range, which was around 80 kilometres away. I packed my skis and travelled there by train. On arrival I discovered there was no snow. Moreover the local army unit knew nothing about a skiing competition. There must have been a serious mix-up. But the result was an enjoyable weekend off with some good friends from medical school serving in the army there – so it wasn't a wasted trip.

7
RYCHNOV NAD KNĚŽNOU, 1959–1962

When I had completed my six months' military service I returned to Nová Paka, this time to work in the Department of Medicine. Thankfully the consultant there was pleasant to deal with, well informed and competent.

In June 1959 I married Olga with whom I had been going out since the second year of our medical studies. We decided to have our wedding lunch at Barandov where there was a convivial restaurant overlooking the river. We did not bother reserving a table, as the party consisted of our four parents and the two of us. But when we arrived we were informed that the restaurant was closed, so we went back to town and had lunch in Mánes, a lovely location overlooking the river and the bridges.

Walking out of the restaurant after our meal we realized that Olga was still grasping an attractive embroidered silk napkin, oblivious to the fact that it should have been left at the table. No one rushed after us to take it back, so she kept it as a memento. As a wedding present from my parents we were given the German equivalent of a jeep. It was a type of Volkswagen called a Kübelwagen. It had 450,000 kilometres on the clock, but it went well. After the war many such vehicles were abandoned at the roadside. People would acquire them and obtain two or three engines from similar old cars. The engine was supported by just four screws, so instead of waiting for a repair the owner would change the engine, take the faulty one to be fixed and carry on driving.

Our honeymoon consisted of five days on the Slapská Dam, where we camped. It was all we could afford at the time, but it was a great holiday.

As I was still determined to specialize in cardiac surgery I applied for a junior doctor's post in the Department of Cardiac Surgery in Hradec Králové. This was a university hospital, part of Charles University and probably the best cardiac surgical department in the country. A few weeks later I received

RYCHNOV NAD KNĚŽNOU, 1959–1962

a letter of acceptance. I was delighted and immediately started planning how to get Olga transferred from Pardubice County to Hradec Králové County in the hope that she, too, might get a post there. It looked promising until she went to the secretariat of the Communist Party in Pardubice to inquire about the progress of her application.

The clerk was not in the office, but she saw on his table a large note saying, 'Do not release Dr [i.e. Mrs] Stark from Pardubice, as her husband will not get the job in Hradec Králové.' We were stunned.

I immediately travelled to Hradec. At a meeting with the representatives of the hospital, the unions and the Communist Party I was told that the job I expected to start within a few weeks had never existed. That was despite the fact that I had received a document stating that I had been accepted for the post.

Not surprisingly, a Communist doctor had left Rychnov and bagged the post in the Department of Cardiac Surgery in Hradec Králové that had originally accepted me. So, despite the fact that I had a confirmation letter in my hands, the promise that I was due to start work there on 1 September meant absolutely nothing. As consolation they told me that I could choose another surgical position in the county.

I discovered that there was a vacancy in Rychnov and Kneznov. I knew that the boss in Rychnov was an outstanding surgeon, so I was glad to accept the position. His name was Dr Jaroslav Kudr, formerly head of abdominal surgery at Hradec University Hospital. He refused to join the military when the hospital was transformed into a military academy, so he was dispatched to Rychnov District Hospital.

Surgically it was great experience for me. The team consisted of four juniors, his deputy and a woman doctor who worked mainly in A&E, one other young man and myself. We would start the day with a ward round before sorting out discharges and admissions. The woman, Dr Pavlová, would then go off to A&E, one of us would attend the fracture clinic, another the urology clinic and another would help out in A&E. So we would not start operating until around noon. Yet, the boss was so dexterous that he could perform a cholecystectomy in twenty minutes and a prostatectomy in thirty minutes. When he did a total gastrectomy he would intubate the patient while one of the nuns acting as anaesthetist would sit with the patient. At the end of the operation he would unscrub and extubate the patient. We did not have an anaesthetist in the department. Our typical operating list consisted of a gastrectomy, two cholecystectomies, an operation for scalenous syndrome or an operation for tennis elbow; the latter had nothing to do with tennis but was the result of repetitive arm movements by blue-collar workers sent to work on assembly lines in factories. Then the list would continue with two or three hernias, a prostatectomy and perhaps an appendectomy or two. So we were probably doing more surgery in one theatre with four juniors and a chief than they were undertaking in the university hospital in Hradec in three theatres with around twenty junior doctors. It was wonderful training, even though I was mostly just assisting.

The chief's deputy was a poor surgeon, but he was considerably more senior than the two newcomers, myself and a Communist doctor. So the boss did not feel he could let me operate. But I still learned a lot. The chief never lost his temper; he was always in control and kind to his staff. One night we were doing a splenectomy for a ruptured spleen on a man who had been caught between two railway wagons. At a crucial moment a scrub nurse known as Big Jarka, during her first night on call, dropped a clamp favoured for use on the splenic artery. Dr Kudr said calmly while pinching the artery with his fingers, 'Don't worry about it, my dear. Just give me any instrument you have.' His attitude and demeanour gave her so much confidence that she developed into an outstanding scrub nurse.

After a few months Olga managed to get a job in paediatrics in a hospital around 30 kilometres from Rychnov. It was another example of how the authorities tried to make life difficult. There were two jobs in paediatrics in Rychnov, yet they posted her to Opočno. I was allocated accommodation sharing one small room with another junior doctor. Olga likewise shared a small room in Opočno with a colleague. So to visit each other for the weekend was only possible when one of those sharing with us went away at the same time.

The orderly in Rychnov's out-patients department was the chairman of the hospital Communist Party. In order to enhance his salary they made him 'senior sister' or charge nurse in the out-patients department despite the fact that he had no nursing training. One Sunday, when I was on call, a young man presented himself with a small wound on his cheek requiring a couple of stitches. Our so-called senior sister Mr Bednář was on duty. He offered to give me a needle holder and a suture, saying that all our sterile towels had been used because we had had a busy weekend. I was not prepared to compromise, so I suggested he call an ambulance to send the patient to the university hospital in Hradec. He was furious, but after a few minutes he provided me with a full sterile table so that I could suture the wound safely.

However, that was not the end of the matter. The next day my chief called me into his office. He said that the hospital director had told him that there had been a complaint about me, that I had been rude to patients. He told the director that he did not believe the allegation as I was never abusive and he had never even heard me swear. But I still had to go to see the director who repeated the accusation to my face. When I asked who had made it he said he could not tell me, as the information had to remain anonymous, but he had no doubt that the allegations were true, as the individual concerned was a trustworthy party member. I said that in that case I had nothing to add, as in my view anonymous accusations were worthless. Next day the director dredged up the subject with my boss yet again. This time my boss, a keen huntsman, said, 'Tell your anonymous informer to be careful because I might empty the entire magazine of my rifle up his arse!'

We generally had to be very careful when a known Communist was around, and of course we did not always know who other informers might be. When I started my job in Rychnov I was advised by the administration that we were not allowed to accept presents from patients apart from cut flowers – up to three stems. When we finished a ward round we would sit in the sister's office. There the nurses would give us milk or coffee and a bread roll or two. This was not allowed. But a nurse was always on guard outside the office to warn us if one of the Communists was approaching.

In autumn 1959 Olga fell pregnant. Visits to each other's hospital became very difficult during the winter, as bus services were poor and driving in our Kübelwagen with its canvass top was cold and unpleasant. She was transferred to Rychnov around Christmas, but we still did not have an apartment of our own. When she went back to work the hospital stoker helped us out. His flat was too big for him – at that time families were allowed only 24 square metres per person plus 12 square metres per family. If you had more you paid extra tax for each metre. If you exceeded your allowance by 50 per cent you could be evicted. So the stoker offered us one of his rooms as a sub-let.

During the winter we went skiing until Olga was about six months pregnant. Then at a routine check they found she was almost completely dilated. She was ordered to go on bed rest, and she spent the next few weeks with her parents in Pardubice. Her friend Dana in Pardubice eventually delivered the baby. At that time I was spending a month learning anaesthesia in the university hospital in Hradec. I will never forget the day Jaroslav was born. I was giving an anaesthetic for a total bladder resection. The urologist was a very slow surgeon, so I popped outside the theatre every forty minutes or so and phoned the Obstetrics Department in Pardubice. After about five hours I got the news. 'It's a boy, and mother and child are doing fine.' I had to continue working for another three hours.

The room in which we lived was just big enough to accommodate a couch for us and a small cot for Jaroslav. There was a wardrobe behind which we placed a double-burner electric stove, on which we prepared infant formula. The hospital's administration could not understand that Olga and I were unable to be on call at the same time, as one of us had to look after the baby. During the day we had a carer, but she lived in the middle of town, while the hospital was on the outskirts, so it was a rush every morning to get him there and for Olga to collect him at four in the afternoon because I was always in theatre. The thorny problem of night calls was eventually settled with the help of my boss who talked to the administrators. Jaroslav spent quite a few hours in the doctors' room in the Department of Paediatrics, where some months later he was happy to sit at the typewriter and bash away at the keys – I have no idea how many typewriters he destroyed. Later on we found another carer, the wife of an ophthalmologist who had two small children and who was willing to look after Jaroslav as well. That was a great relief.

Generally I was lucky with the car and its maintenance. A brother of our ward sister was a car mechanic. He was something of a hypochondriac, constantly asking me for advice and for prescriptions. Consequently he was very happy to repair our vehicle and keep it on the road. As he lived in a village near by this was easy. If anything went wrong I would drive the car there, and in no time he would fix the problem.

Early one Monday morning we were driving with Olga from Prague to Rychnov. Suddenly without warning the car ground to a halt. I did not know what to do. Eventually we stopped a lorry and asked the driver for help. Straight away he asked if we had petrol. I assured him that we had. So he checked everything under the bonnet but not having identified the problem he enquired once more about the fuel levels. The car had no petrol gauge. We simply opened the filling tap and prodded a wooden stick into the reservoir. With no explanation for our problem, he did this and – surprise, surprise – it was empty.

In 1962 Olga applied to the hospital director to sit an examination in paediatrics, but he did not provide her with a recommendation because of some minor dispute they had had not long before. This had consequences. Her chief did not turn up for work one day. He was living with his family in Pardubice and commuted the 40 kilometres to Rychnov for the week, returning home at weekends. When he did not come one Monday everyone at the hospital thought that he had stayed at home, perhaps with a cold or other minor illness. In fact he had been arrested that morning on his way to work. It turned out that his ageing father used to meet regularly with friends, and, as evangelists, they sang religious hymns. Although Olga's boss was not involved in these activities he had been arrested.

So suddenly there was a crisis in the Department of Paediatrics. The hospital director asked Olga to be locum head of department. Olga said that she could not take on this role as she had not taken the paediatrics examination, but my boss, Dr Kudr, had a word with her assuring her of his full support. He felt it would be better not to antagonize the administration. But he promised that if any problem arose he would take full responsibility.

So just three and half years after graduation she became a consultant. And when I was on call – we surgeons covered paediatrics – she was my boss. As soon as Olga accepted her senior position she asked for an apartment. Three of us living in one room was proving difficult, so the director promised to get us a flat within two months – that is, before the end of the year. If she did not get the accommodation it was agreed that she could resign her position. I think the administration did not take the matter very seriously, so when Olga went to see the hospital director he was taken aback. It was 29 December, one day before the deadline. He stormed off to the offices of the local council, swearing all the way. Miraculously, the next day we had a flat large enough for all of us, and Olga's Aunt Olda helped look after Jaroslav.

In 1963 a research post was advertised in the Department of Paediatric Surgery in Prague. It was *aspirantura* – a three-year research post to complete a C.Sc. thesis (the equivalent of Ph.D.) in the cardiac subdivision. Olga was supportive, as I had always wanted to specialize in paediatric cardiac surgery, and by then I was twenty-nine. The interview was tough. I thought that I did not answer all the questions satisfactorily, and Dr Padovcova, head of paediatric cardiology, came up with the most difficult ones. Fortunately I passed and was accepted for the post. Later on we became personal friends, and when we moved to London she visited us a few times.

The next hurdle was to be released from Rychnov. Although my chief, or *primář*, was supportive I knew the hospital was not keen to let me go, but we also knew that Olga could leave her post any time, as Jaroslav was still an infant. We checked in Prague at the doctors' union headquarters, and the law was clear. So we decided to play a game with the hospital administration.

The hospital needed Olga badly because she was still locum consultant following the arrest of her chief. We had a meeting with the hospital director as well as the Communist Party and the union's representatives. When my request for release from Rychnov was turned down Olga calmly stated that she intended to stop working from the following month. When they asked why she said that bringing up a child as a good member of society was her first duty, to which the director replied that he understood. He said, 'Look how I failed with my own daughter! She became a single mother.' At this point the union representative said that under a special law doctors could not leave their jobs to look after their children.

Olga produced a letter from the union's headquarters in Prague confirming that mothers of young children, in whatever profession, could stay at home. After some further discussion they agreed to release me, providing Olga would stay until the following June. That was eight months ahead, but we thought that this would be manageable. So I moved to Prague to live with my parents, and Olga remained with Jaroslav in Rychnov. Fortunately her Aunt Olda was available to stay to assist with child care.

8
PRAGUE, 1963–1965

In September 1963 I started work at the university Department of Paediatric Surgery in Prague, by far the youngest member of the team. I participated in everything, attending out-patients, working on the ward and in theatre. In theatre I would assist, occasionally operating on a hernia or an appendix. All the juniors rotated, administering anaesthesia and working as scrub nurses. It was useful experience, but ultimately I was disappointed. None of the surgeons came close to displaying the surgical skills of Primář Kudr from Rychnov. I remember one day assisting Dr Frank in an oesophageal replacement by colon that took twelve hours. A few years later David Waterston in London performed the same operation in ninety minutes.

Starting my thesis was on my mind. The subject suggested by Dr Padovcova, head of Paediatric Cardiology, was 'Validation of Carbon Dioxide Values Obtained by Rebreathing Technique Compared with Direct Blood Measurements'. The reason she suggested the topic was our lack of equipment. Instead of taking blood samples and measuring on the Astrup machine we had to do rebreathing. I spent hours learning rebreathing, then learning how to work an Astrup machine. So I was running between our Surgical Department, the Department of Respiratory Medicine and the Physiology Laboratory. After around twelve months Dr Šamánek from the Department of Paediatric Cardiology left for a scholarship in Philadelphia. I was asked by the cardiologists to dissect the saphenous vein when they catheterized a child. Before this only Dr Šamánek was deemed sufficiently well trained to undertake this procedure. I struck a bargain. I said that I would be happy to dissect the vein for them, but in return they must teach me the basic techniques of cardiac catheterization. And they did, so, years later, when cases were presented in London at our Joint Cardiac Conference I was able to enquire knowledgeably as to which type of catheter cardiologists had used.

47

The following year there was another vacancy for an 'aspirant' in our department. I suggested my good friend Bohouš Hučín who was working in Vlašim, south of Prague, to our chief, Professor Kafka. Bohouš was appointed, and soon I had a kindred spirit – two young medics working with ageing male and female doctors.

In January 1965 an American professor, a friend of Professor Kafka, came on sabbatical to visit our department. The day before he arrived the professor asked who would like to interpret during the radiology round next morning when we would be examining X-rays of our patients with the radiologists. As nobody volunteered I offered my services, even though I was the most junior member of the team. After the ward round he asked if I would like to take his guests, Professor Kiesewetter and his wife, on a sightseeing tour of Prague in my car. As already mentioned, it was a somewhat unusual vehicle: a German version of a jeep called a Kübelwagen.

So I took our visitors on a sightseeing tour of the city, which they enjoyed greatly. The Kübelwagen was clearly extraordinary in their eyes and a big hit. That evening Professor Kafka invited us all to Klášterní Vinárna, a good restaurant near the National Theatre. During the meal Professor Kiesewetter asked me where outside Czechoslovakia I had trained. I laughed and explained that, living in a Communist state, we were not allowed to go anywhere. So he suggested a one-year fellowship in his department in Pittsburgh. Almost immediately he realized his error: the USA was unlikely to be regarded as an acceptable nation for a professional exchange to the Czech authorities. However, since he was continuing his sabbatical in the UK he suggested I come to work at Great Ormond Street Hospital instead. This was regarded as a Mecca for paediatric cardiac surgery, so I agreed with alacrity.

I thought all this idle chat over a bottle of red wine and did not expect anything to come of it. Our visitors left Czechoslovakia the next day, but the following week Professor Kafka was flying to Edinburgh to attend the meeting of the British Association of Paediatric Surgeons. I was sure that Mr David Waterston from Great Ormond Street Hospital would be there, so before he flew out I asked him to enquire about the possibility of my spending time at his hospital. He said, 'Certainly. But as you know I am very forgetful, so please give me ten notes saying 'Ask re Stark – Great Ormond Street' before I go. I'll put them in with my socks, in my underpants and with my shirts.'

The next day he left. When he returned ten days later he did not say a word on the subject when he turned up for the ward round. I felt that that was the end of the matter, but at the end of the round I went into his office and enquired. He told me I had been offered a job for a month. He added, 'You'll have to write to the consultants in London and explain that you will not be allowed to take any currency out of the country. Your British hosts will have to pay for everything.' I spent the next two days with my English teacher trying to compose a suitable letter explaining my predicament while expressing my profound appreciation for the London surgeons' offer of such a wonderful opportunity to extend my knowledge.

On the third day a cable arrived from the UK. I had been offered a job as a senior registrar for a month on full pay with free accommodation. Olga was extremely supportive, although our domestic situation in Prague was problematic. We were living with my parents, and although we had made some structural alterations to separate their flat into two units there was little privacy. It was the apartment in which I had grown up and where my father had his surgery. We had blocked the door from the waiting-room to his surgery, which now became our main living-room as well as bedroom. The little corridor between the surgery and the second surgery where his assistant sometimes worked was converted into a bathroom, and the second surgery became Jaroslav's room. We shared the kitchen with my mother. When the day came to leave for London, Olga accompanied me to the main railway station. She asked, 'What will you do if they offer you an extension of the post?' I thought it was extremely unlikely, so I didn't give this a second thought.

9
LONDON, 1965–1967

Because I was unsure whether I would be allowed to travel to the West ever again I bought a train ticket that would take me to London via Brussels, where I spent the night tramping the city on foot, absorbing the sights. I was not allowed to change any money. All I had was a five-pound note bought in Prague on the black market. I worried how to get it across the border, but my father had a suggestion: place it in a condom and insert it into a tube of toothpaste. He thought it would be safe there. And so it was.

When I arrived in London I took the Underground train to Holborn and, as instructed, walked up Southampton Row across Queen Square to Great Ormond Street. I walked into the first hospital along the street and asked for David Waterston. I was in the wrong place; it was the Royal London Homoeopathic Hospital. Eventually I located the correct hospital, which was next door.

I was swiftly provided with accommodation in a small room in the adjoining residential quarters, but I got a shock the next morning when there was a brisk knock on the door. I was fast asleep, as I had spent the whole of the previous night walking around Brussels. It was a maid with a tray of tea. With a broad smile she said, 'Good morning, sir. Your morning tea.' It was quite unlike Communist Czechoslovakia.

Shortly after I went downstairs to the residents' mess for breakfast. I ate alone. Nobody said a word to me. Some individuals were reading newspapers next to their plates, others just sat quietly eating. My first thought was: How can they tell I'm from Czechoslovakia? Are they ignoring me? Yet as soon as we walked out of the mess and began heading down a lengthy corridor to the hospital they immediately became friendly, chatting to me like old friends. I learned that in England during breakfast most people don't talk. One reads one's daily paper and minds one's own business. But the

LONDON, 1965–1967

Europeans' popular perception of the 'cold Englishman' was completely false. Maybe one reason for the friendliness of my junior colleagues, as well as the consultants, was the fact that Great Ormond Street was such an international hospital, with personnel arriving to work there from all over the world. About a third of the consultants were from abroad. As I was to discover later, the atmosphere in some of the older teaching hospitals was markedly different.

I had no language problems at first. In general I understood the English spoken around me pretty well. Iain Aberdeen, one of my two consultants, was an exception. He was Australian, and when he got excited in theatre – which was often – and started shouting behind his mask I could not make out a word he was saying. I had further problems on the telephone. When I was on call and a nurse phoned to ask if she could give a child an aspirin, for instance, I had to get up, dress and walk over to the ward to get clarification. Understanding people on the phone proved a particular challenge at first, especially as the hospital employed nurses from all over Britain with their broad regional accents: Geordies from the far north of England, Welsh, Scots, Cornish and others whose speech patterns were unfamiliar to me.

Around the third day after my arrival I was having coffee in the surgeons' room next to the theatres with the second senior registrar Subramanian, nicknamed Subra, a huge Indian fellow, when Mr Waterston, our senior consultant, walked in. Subra said, 'David, Jarda could stay for a whole year, you know, not just for a month.' To which the consultant responded, in his characteristically slow and deliberate fashion, 'How wonderful.' And he meant it. That was how my stay was extended to a year.

In my excitement I phoned Olga in Prague explaining what a fantastic opportunity this was. She sportingly agreed and said she would try to get my stay extended via the Czech authorities. This was very generous-spirited of her. When I was away in London she had to live with our son in my parents' flat in Prague. My father was not particularly keen on my choice of Olga as my spouse, as he felt that a wife should stay at home and look after the children, not go out to work. He was rather old-fashioned in such matters.

Professor Kafka also agreed to the extension of my stay, but the bureaucracy that had to be faced was a nightmare. It was necessary to get formal permission from all the university authorities and from the corresponding offices of the Communist Party. Over the next four to five months Olga became very familiar with all the old palaces in Malá Strana, an historic quarter of

Prague where most of the ministries' offices were located. At one stage things looked bleak. Somehow my papers got lost, and she was told that if I did not return to Prague within a week I would be considered an illegal emigrant.

It was probably fortunate that when the offer of a temporary post at Great Ormond Street was made I did not know what the position of senior registrar involved. In Prague I was the most junior member of the team, although as an 'aspirant' my role was slightly modified. I was supposed to undertake my research and do clinical work on the side, so my workload was not generally too arduous. In London a senior registrar was the most senior junior doctor under the consultant. Subra was far more experienced, and I was on call all the time, except for Wednesday afternoons and nights, so he would cover me and provide advice. We called consultants only when we had to take a child to theatre. If it was something reasonably simple and the consultant trusted us, he would tell us to go ahead and we would take charge of the operation. Otherwise one of us would open the chest and the consultant would arrive to undertake the surgery. The senior registrar had to ensure the smooth running of the unit, set up operating lists, organize post-operative care and so on. So I am not sure whether if I had known what I was letting myself in for I would have come to London at all. I think I would. The work was very hard but the training incredibly good. We also had to give a number of lectures at the hospital.

My annual salary was £800, with free accommodation and meals. Taking into account the fiscal exchange rate between the UK and Czechoslovakia, it was a fortune. I was careful not to spend much while abroad, and on my return home Olga was able to buy a Fiat 600 in Tuzex – a special shop selling goods only for foreign hard currency.

Early on during my time in London Amrit Darjee, an Indian house surgeon from South Africa, suggested that he and I take a long weekend and drive to Cornwall. He had a small Mini. On Friday Violet, the head waitress in the doctors' mess, handed each of us a brown paper bag. 'You impoverished doctors will need something for the weekend' was all she said. In each bag we found a pack of butter, some cuts of cold meat, cheese, carrots and masses of fruit. We collected Amrit's girlfriend and set off. We drove to Devon and Cornwall. I still remember staying in a B&B in Mevagissey, a lovely little harbour town. Apart from this trip most of the time we were tied to Great Ormond Street, so the weekend away was both enjoyable and memorable.

LONDON, 1965–1967

While in London I became very friendly with Mike Tynan, who was a medical (cardiology) registrar. We spent a lot of time working and writing medical papers together – usually in my flat at Great Ormond Street. I remember one day we were discussing a paper and I made some coffee. Mike was delighted – he'd never had such a good cup of coffee before. 'How do you make it?' he asked. As I showed him, his eyes grew bigger and bigger. He informed me that the amount of coffee I had used for the two of us would probably have lasted him a whole week. I later learned something from him about making tea. His method involved around three or four times more tea than I would have used in Prague.

Before Christmas it was traditional for the junior doctors and the nurses and secretaries to put on a seasonal show. It would be rehearsed for weeks. Terry Mahon, Dr Gerald Graham's secretary, was very much the impresario. Dr Graham was a cardiologist and in charge of the heart–lung machine. I was asked to recite Hamlet's 'To be or not to be' soliloquy in Czech. I was told it was a great success. Another sketch was called 'Mirror, Mirror on the Wall, Can You Tell Me . . .' Professor Wilkinson, a general paediatric surgeon, was known not to be a very good technical surgeon. So in an obvious allusion to him, the cast chanted, 'Mirror, mirror on the wall, can you tell me . . . Do I know how to operate?' And the chorus came back: 'NO!' It seemed amazing get away with making fun of their consultants and how this was accepted in good humour.

During that first Christmas in London I was asked to dinner on Christmas Day by Corrie, Subra's Norwegian wife. She also invited Willy Krauthamer from Switzerland, a young doctor working in the Electroencephalogram or EEG Department. He had far more difficulty with the English language than I did. When Corrie served up the turkey she asked him which part of the bird he would like. Willy got very excited and replied, 'Oh, I love stiff breasts!' His *faux pas* was repeated around the hospital for quite some time.

In the meantime the family situation in Prague was increasingly tense. My mother had agreed to look after our son because Olga was still working. But my father maintained that my mother was in the process of looking for a job, so we should pay her to undertake child care. Although this was probably against my mother's wishes, we agreed to this arrangement and paid her a monthly wage from then on, although I suspected that my mother was more than happy to look after Jaroslav and that she had no intention of seeking paid work elsewhere. But when Olga was presented with a bill for every ice cream or banana my mother bought Jaroslav my wife was not happy. So I felt guilty leaving her in Prague with my not especially supportive parents. On the other hand, I had to remind myself that it was a wonderful opportunity to work at Great Ormond Street, not only for myself but for the family, both professionally and financially.

My consultants in London asked me if I would stay for another year, as Subra was heading off to do research in the USA. Olga – wonderful as ever – and my professor were in favour of such an extension. But Professor Máček, the dean of the Medical School in Prague, wrote to me saying I should return and finish my thesis and only then would they allow me to go back to London. Undoubtedly he had no idea what a prestigious position being senior registrar at Great Ormond Street was. There were usually thirty or so applicants for one such position from all over the world, so I would have no chance of securing the post again once I returned to Czechoslovakia. Eventually Professor Kafka managed to persuade the dean that the extension was for the best – and long-suffering Olga once more started running from one Prague office to another to secure my stay in the West.

Olga approached our neighbour Mr Šebor. He was a pre-war Communist idealist who appreciated what a unique opportunity it was to work in one of the best departments of paediatric cardiac surgery in the world; an opportunity not just for me but of long-term benefit to the country. He also felt in my debt, as I had looked after his son after a heart operation when I was working in the Intensive Therapy Unit in Prague. He used to work for the Ministry of Education, which had issued my original passport, and also for the Ministry of Foreign Affairs, which was supposed to extend my exit visa or else issue a new passport. He went to the clerk in charge of sending telegrams and instructed him to cable the London Embassy saying that my stay had been extended for a year and that they should amend my passport duly. The clerk was unwilling but finally agreed, as he had known Mr Šebor for years. So my exit visa was extended on the basis of his cable, and my position was secure.

Getting my family over to London for visits was not easy. Once Olga came for a month, then my father arrived with young Jaroslav for two weeks. The policy was not to allow the entire family over together in order to ensure that I would return to Czechoslovakia in due course. Olga and I would have loved her to have accompanied Jaroslav. But initially there seemed no chance of this. She discussed it with Mr Šebor who said he would do his best to see if it were possible but required assurances that we would all eventually return. If we had emigrated as a family he would have been in terrible trouble. Olga gave him her word, although she knew that my ambition was to stay in the UK on a permanent basis.

The good news came that she had been granted an exit visa valid for two months. She packed our Fiat 600 and drove across Europe with Jaroslav, aged seven, taking charge of navigation all the way. On arrival we enrolled him at the local school, St George's, in Queen Square, where he generally got on very well. Shortly after they arrived Alena Lehovská turned up with her son Honza. Her husband Miloš was working for a year with Dr Pampiglione in the EEG Department at Great Ormond Street. Alena had been in the same year at medical school as Olga and me. In fact she had been born a day earlier then me in the same obstetric hospital – and our mothers were in the same room. We ski'ed with them on several occasions, so we remained good friends over the years. One day Jaroslav and Honza came home from school, and Honza, who was a year younger than our son, said Jaroslav had been 'great' at school. When we asked what he meant by this he told us that the pupils sometimes singled them out as foreigners and were unpleasant to them. But Jaroslav had found a solution. During school breaks, when they were out in the playground, the two friends would stand with their backs to a wall and if any student approached them aggressively they would kick out. This was how they defended themselves against the school bullies.

We were given an apartment at Great Ormond Street for junior doctors with families. It was in a very old, rather decrepit building, but to us it was a palace. In the UK there was a rule that children under a certain age must not be left at home on their own. One evening, when friends had invited Olga and me to dinner, we started to discuss child-care arrangements. Jaroslav overheard and said adamantly, 'I am *not* having a babysitter. You're welcome to go out, but if you're thinking of calling a babysitter you're going nowhere!' That was it. He was so resolute about us not calling in a stranger to mind him that we left him by himself for a few hours, and he was perfectly happy. Some months later we drove up together to Stratford-upon-Avon to see Shakespeare's *Coriolanus*. It was a very long play, so we expected Jaroslav to be fast asleep by the time we returned to our B&B in Stratford. But, no, he had read somewhere about Leonardo da Vinci's 'secret writing'. The artist apparently wrote against a mirror so the letters were hard to decipher. Jaroslav was absorbed in doing his own version of Leonardo's writing while we were out watching the play.

We decided to take our summer holiday in France and Italy because we were not sure if we would be able to do something like this once we returned to Prague. We packed the Fiat, borrowed a roof rack to which we strapped our tent – and off we went. We drove right through France. The day we went to see Chartres Cathedral Jaroslav preferred to stay in the car reading his comics. We continued down to the French Riviera, then to Italy: Genoa, Florence, Rome and all the way to Sorrento. It was a wonderful holiday, but camping could be hard work; however, we didn't have much money to spend. In Florence we went out for dinner to a little trattoria. Jaroslav was fond of milk, so he asked for a glass with his meal, but when we discovered that it was far more expensive than wine he got a glass of wine! We were determined to see as much of France and Italy as possible. And we did so in those three memorable weeks.

Eventually Olga and Jaroslav returned to Prague, while I had another six weeks to complete at Great Ormond Street before flying home. Just before they left we received a letter from my parents telling us that they had exchanged their apartment in Pařížská Street for a smaller one on Bethlehem Square. This came as a shock, as it included our accommodation as well. We had built the partition, furnished our two rooms and spent a lot of time and energy making it our home.

My mother and father had packed our furniture and effects into boxes and placed them in storage. When Olga and Jaroslav returned to Prague they had nowhere to live. With the help of some friends Olga found a sub-let in Břevnov on the outskirts of Prague consisting of a single room with a tap in the corridor for washing. My parents' rationale to us was that the exchange of flats was such a wonderful opportunity they could not let it go. I so was shocked by their lack of concern for our welfare I never forgave them.

When I arrived at the main railway station in Prague a month and a half later I was shamefaced when they checked my luggage at customs. In fact I think the customs officer was more embarrassed than me. I had packed at the last minute, as I had been on duty until very late, so I had thrown everything into the suitcase without thought: dirty underpants and smelly socks all jumbled up with the scientific reprints and the presents I was bringing home.

10
BACK IN PRAGUE, 1968

I joined Olga and Jaroslav in the single room in which they were now forced to live. I had to defend my C.Sc. thesis. This was scheduled to take place in the lecture theatre of the Orthopaedic Surgery Clinic of Professor Hněvkovský. It was well received, but a female professor of paediatrics from Slovakia objected to the fact that my transparencies had English captions and annotations. 'Demonstrates not enough concern for your mother tongue,' she pronounced. The fact that I had written the thesis in London did not cut much ice. But at the age of thirty-four I got my degree – and I could now put C.Sc. after my name.

Writing the thesis in London had not been easy. I had very little free time, and as it had to be in Czech I dictated it into a Dictaphone and took the tapes to the Czech Embassy where a sympathetic secretary typed up the text for me. I then sent sections by post to Olga – who was always the best editor of my scientific papers. She corrected not only my Czech, which I knew was not very good, but also the scientific content with which she was less familiar. So drafts were flying backwards and forwards with a lot of exclamation marks and expletives – but the important thing was that the thesis had been completed and submitted.

As was customary I had to provide refreshments and alcohol after I had presented my thesis. I had two bottles of Black and White whisky, but clearly it would not be enough for us all. So I went downstairs to the neighbouring building where there was a convenience store and bought a few bottles of Blue Portugal red wine. At the time it was considered a reasonably good wine, but basically it was plonk. So mixing it with whisky was lethal. By the time we got home I was not only drunk but very sick, so our main concern was to hide my condition from Jaroslav – which we somehow managed to do.

I started working at my old hospital Na Karlově in paediatric surgery.

Until I returned from the UK I did not know whether I would be taken on as a houseman, an assistant (the equivalent of a senior registrar) or in some other capacity. As the head of Cardiac Surgery, Docent Brodský, had left to work for a year in Sweden a few days before my arrival I found myself locum head of Cardiac Surgery. It was exciting but not easy. We did not have a heart–lung machine, so we could do only closed heart surgery.

One of my first cases was a four-year-old 'blue baby'. One Friday afternoon I was asked to see a patient in the Cardiology Department across the street. The patient was a four-year-old girl with Fallot's tetralogy; she was very blue and squatting almost all the time. The cardiologist, Dr Voříšková, pleaded with me to put the child on the Monday operating list. But that was not what I had learned from my years in London. I was firm. 'We have to operate now.' I went back to our department and talked to the theatre sister on call saying we had an emergency. She asked if it was an incarcerated hernia or an appendix. I replied no, it was a Blalock–Taussig shunt. She was horrified. 'But that's not an emergency. It's cardiac surgery!' Eventually she relented, and we prepared to operate. One problem was that we did not have suitably small cardiovascular clamps. I knew that they had them in IKEM, a prestigious adult cardiac centre in Krč. This department was full of high-powered Communist surgeons; therefore their equipment was first class. I phoned them and asked if I could borrow a couple of Castaneda clamps for a few hours. They agreed, so I took my Fiat, drove to Krč, borrowed the clamps, returned to our hospital, performed the Blalock–Taussig shunt procedure and drove back to Krč with the clamps. It was very different from London.

Around June we got our own apartment. It was a *Družstevní byt* or cooperative flat paid for by my parents-in-law. They had inherited and sold a house near Pardubice and given us the money. It was in a high-rise building in the Pankrác district, and to us it was heaven; we had a living area and two bedrooms. The one drawback was the lack of a telephone. This is why I had to sleep in the hospital each time I operated on a cardiac patient. Another problem was our on-call rota. I was on the rota for 'assistants' (senior registrars), which comprised five senior surgeons, none of whom was trained in cardiac surgery. So on the days I operated I would secretly stay in the hospital. From about five in the afternoon to around midnight I would skulk in my small room so as not to be seen or upset anyone in charge. The nurses knew that they could call me if there were complications. About midnight I went down to the Resuscitation Unit (the Intensive Care Unit), examined the patients, adjusted their medication and went to bed.

This is how things were before that summer in 1968 when we went off camping on the isle of Veli Lošinj in Yugoslavia all too aware of the tense political situation back home.

Dubček, First Secretary of the Communist Party, had been appointed the previous December. His was the most prestigious political position in the country, higher than that of a president or a prime minister. Although he was a Communist he was an idealist who wanted to implement 'socialism with a human face'. At that time this seemed to be our best chance of development and progress. A vote for anyone else would likely lead to a Soviet invasion. We were unsure what to do. Should we vote for a Communist? As things turned out, we never had to make that decision.

We returned from our holidays less than twenty-four hours before the Warsaw Pact armies invaded our homeland. When Olga called her parents, her mother said that she had been woken up by her husband telling her to get up – as the entire Russian Army had come to congratulate her on her birthday!

11
LONDON, 1968–1970

So Olga, Jaroslav and I arrived in London in our little car. There was no suitable vacancy at Great Ormond Street, as it was the wrong time of year to apply. My former consultants very kindly created a research job for me at the Institute of Child Health, an academic department of the hospital. Because no hospital accommodation was available Iain Aberdeen generously invited us to stay at his house in Highgate, where we remained for six weeks until a hospital flat came free. It was only by chance some ten years later that I learned that two consultants had paid my salary out of their own pockets during my eight months' research. They sent the money to the hospital, so I received a payslip every month and had no idea of their kindness. I do not think this would happen in many other countries. So much for the perception of the British as cold and reserved.

My research involved examining the influence of suture techniques and material on the growth of the aorta, which was relevant to surgery for coarctation of the aorta. I operated on one or two piglets a week. We would kill the pigs at regular intervals after surgery, look at the aortic growth and obtain specimens for histology. This meant we ate at least one piglet for dinner a week. We had to devise a special technique for killing them, as we discovered that those killed by thiopentone overdose tasted dreadful. Olga and I experimented with different recipes to ring the changes; the ones involving oregano were the most successful.

The following spring I wished to attend the American College of Cardiology meeting in Dallas, where my paper had been accepted. As I had been using Ethicon sutures in my experiments, I tried to get some backing from the company. The Ethicon representative invited me to a lunch at the Savoy Grill, so I was optimistic about receiving substantial financial support. We had a good lunch, and he wrote me out a cheque for £10 and asked if I would be willing to visit the plant in New Jersey to give a lecture. I was bitterly disappointed, as I needed considerably more than this for a trip to Texas.

I attended the Dallas meeting anyway. I stayed in a small cheap hotel, and the afternoon after my arrival I went for a walk, mainly to establish where the conference hotel was situated and where I had to go the following morning. All of a sudden I found myself in the midst of a shoot-out. I was unsure what to do. Lie down? Run? I stayed put. After about five minutes the shooting stopped and I walked back to my accommodation. The next day there were huge headlines in the local newspapers: 'Burglary in a Jewelry Store. Three Policemen Severely Wounded'. When I arrived at the meeting and told my American friends what had happened they looked at me in disbelief and exclaimed, 'Jarda, you're a fool. If you feel like going for a walk, take a taxi instead!'

I attended the meeting with Mike Tynan and Ian Carr, a very bright British Heart Foundation cardiology fellow. At the meeting we projected each other's slides, not trusting the official projectionist not to mix them up.

In 1969 I also attended meetings in Colmar, where I presented two papers in French, as well as one in Belfast and another in Dublin.

When I finished my research I was appointed a fellow or senior registrar at Great Ormond Street for a year. It was a fantastic experience, as I became familiar with all the surgical techniques and thoroughly enjoyed surgery, running an operating list and having overall responsibility for post-operative care. I was on call most of the time, but this was no hardship. Jaroslav was having a good time at school, and Olga, too, was getting job satisfaction working for Alistair Dudgeon, the head of the Department of Microbiology. She was involved in the rubella register, working closely with Catherine Peckham who later became renowned in this field.

One day the famous American surgeon Dr John Kirklin visited our unit. He was regarded as the father of cardiac surgery – in many people's opinion he was a god. When he arrived at the theatre suite Danny, our Thai orderly, was the only member of staff outside the theatre. Dr Kirklin asked him how the operation was progressing, and Danny replied gravely, 'Very well! Mr Aberdeen has just located the heart.'

It was a tradition at the hospital to hold a dinner party once a month to welcome new junior doctors and say goodbye to those who were leaving. Formal dress was required. The hospital provided food; we paid only for drinks. I still recall the first such dinner Olga and I attended that year. We were sitting in a remote corner, and it was hard for the waitresses to serve us. In front of us were six wine glasses, and we had no idea which was meant for what. When the waitress came to serve the first wine we did not know which glasses to pass over to her, which was embarrassing, since it was such a formal and traditionally British occasion – but after a few drinks we quickly forgot our *faux pas*.

The Boat Race, the traditional rowing contest between Oxford and Cambridge universities, takes place on the Thames between Putney and Mortlake in London each April. People have picnics along the banks of the river and enjoy the thrill when the university they support wins. One year we went with Jack and Beth Cahill and their children. Jack was an American, a fellow senior registrar with me at Great Ormond Street, and our two families had a memorable day out together.

In 1970 it was clear to me that there was very little prospect of obtaining a job in paediatric cardiac surgery in the UK, as there were only four full-time paediatric cardiac surgeons in the whole country and no new posts were being created. The consultants I worked for suggested that I go to the USA to undertake research and become known there. As I had been very well trained by them they expected that someone would offer me an appropriately good job in North America. The first hurdle was to pass the Educational Certificate for Foreign Medical Graduates (ECFMG) examination, which was a requirement to work in the USA. Most of my colleagues had taken this soon after graduation when the scientific disciplines of chemistry, physiology and so on were still fresh in their minds. I had graduated twelve years earlier, after which I had worked in general and paediatric cardiac surgery, so my knowledge of the basics was long forgotten. With some trepidation I did some reading but not that much, as most of the time I was working or on call. At any rate I sat the examination and managed somehow to get through.

The second hurdle was requalification. I was working via a temporary licence, which had been granted to me as a graduate of Charles University in Prague, but my degree would not have been accepted as valid if I wanted to work permanently in the UK, as there was no reciprocity between Charles University and UK medical institutions. I knew, however, that I could work on temporary registration indefinitely. The Medical Council had told me when I went for my usual annual extension that they would extend it indefinitely but that I must never tell them I intended to remain permanently in the UK. The temporary registration was meant to be temporary.

I realized that if I wanted to come back from the USA and apply for a consultant post I had better get a degree from the UK. This was a much more difficult undertaking than the ECFMG examination. All the bodies granting full registration required an examination in internal medicine, surgery, gynaecology and obstetrics and pathology. Pathology included microbiology, pathology and histology. It was an intimidating prospect. Fortunately there was one institution, Apothecaries' Hall in Dublin, that did not require pathology. So, although it was looked on as a second-class degree, I decided to go for that one. For around six months I spent my free Wednesday afternoons at University College Hospital learning obstetrics and gynaecology, because I did not have a clue how to examine pregnant mothers. I spent a few of my Wednesdays at St Bartholomew's Hospital where I brushed up on neurology and diabetes. Finally I was ready to go to Dublin. I obtained accommodation with a very welcoming family in that city through a contact at Great Ormond Street. They were Protestants living in the mainly Catholic Republic of Ireland who said they felt very much in the minority and even, at times, like outcasts. They made me aware for the first time of the problems that can be caused by religious as well as political differences. I got on with them well, and everyone in the household was very kind to me.

I had to do four examinations. In addition to clinical subjects I had to learn how to make pills, since my degree was being awarded by the Apothecaries' Hall. Each examination was separated by a week's interval, and one had to pass all four. If one failed one it was necessary to wait another six months for the next examination date and do all four again. So for the first time I found myself under considerable stress. My family and I were supposed to fly to Boston on 1 July, but because of my examinations we delayed travelling until mid-August. In Dublin I was frantically trying to relearn long-forgotten subjects and do an examination on them – and immediately relearn something else.

Eddie Tempany worked as a paediatrician at Dublin's Children's Hospital, and Barry O'Donnell was a general paediatric surgeon who operated on some simpler heart conditions as well. They invited me one weekend to join them at the local yacht club for lunch and offered their professional support. I have a feeling they mentioned my name to the examiners. When I did a practical case in my medicine examination my patient was a young woman with asthma. Everything seemed crystal clear, but I had been warned in advance not to start by telling examiners the diagnosis – merely to describe the symptoms and signs. So I did so, and the examiner asked, 'Well, do you know the diagnosis?' I repeated the symptoms and signs, and he seemed irritated. 'Do you know the diagnosis or not?' So I said yes I did but that I had been told never to mention it in this kind of examination. He laughed and showed me the patient's electrocardiogram. He must have been aware that I worked in the cardiac unit at Great Ormond Street; otherwise he would not have expected a candidate for a basic medical degree to know much about ECGs. I described how I interpreted it, and he was happy to pass me.

After four weeks I was a Licensee of Apothecaries' Hall (LAH), allowed to practise medicine in the UK and Ireland. As an added bonus I could run a pharmacy in Ireland! Some years later, after I became a consultant, I was looking after a very sick private patient in the Harley Street Clinic postoperatively. Sadly the patient died in the early hours of the morning. I filled in the death certificate, a procedure usually undertaken by my registrar, and went home to catch a few hours' sleep. Around ten o'clock in the morning Barbara, the head nurse from the Intensive Therapy Unit, informed me that the coroner wanted to talk to me. She gave me his phone number, and I called him. He asked me if I was a qualified doctor as he had never come across the letters 'LAH'. I explained what they signified, but he seemed doubtful. Only when I told him that I was a senior cardiac surgeon at Great Ormond Street was he happy to accept the validity of my qualification.

A week after I returned from Dublin to London David Waterston told me that they were looking for a paediatric cardiac surgeon at the Royal Postgraduate Medical School at Hammersmith Hospital. The post had been advertised, and they had asked him if he knew somebody suitable for the post. The stumbling block was that they wanted someone who would develop a first-class infant cardiac surgery unit but who could also work as a general paediatric surgeon, undertaking occasional neurosurgery and paediatric orthopaedics. Mr Waterston told Professor Hugh Bentall that the training of a cardiac surgeon in the UK did not involve doing general paediatric surgery or paediatric orthopaedics but there was one person with the qualifications they were after – and that person was Jarda Stark.

Olga and I were not especially keen to emigrate once more, so the prospect of a job at Hammersmith Hospital was an attractive one. I was invited to visit and enquired about the closing date for applications. I was informed that it had officially closed a week earlier but that that should pose no problem. I duly left my application with them.

I thought I had better make some enquiries before I went much further. How many operating sessions would I have? The answer I received was rather odd. 'We understand that most infant cardiac surgery is done at night so you would not need a regular session.' Next I asked how many beds I would have? 'Well, we all share beds so you do not need any of your own.' It was all a bit disheartening, but I went for the interview since I had been shortlisted. The only other candidate was an Indian fellow from Manchester who had done some paediatric urology but undertaken no cardiac surgery at all.

The committee was heavily weighted in my favour. My boss David Waterston represented the Royal College of Surgeons, a Great Ormond Street surgeon called Harold Nixon was there for the region and Herbert Epstein, also a general surgeon at Great Ormond Street, represented another professional body. During the interview I could not help but repeat my concerns. I told the committee that I did not think that developing a first-class infant cardiac surgical unit in 1970 was compatible with undertaking occasional general, orthopaedic and neurosurgery.

In the end the committee recommended that the Hammersmith Hospital should reconsider its job description and readvertise the post. Some two years later I talked to Chris Lincoln, a fellow senior registrar from Great Ormond Street and a good friend, who said he had attended a dinner party given by Professor Selwyn Taylor, the dean of Hammersmith Hospital, during which Professor Taylor mentioned that a while before he had attended an interview where the applicant had interviewed the committee rather than the other way round. Chris guessed he was referring to me.

12
BOSTON, 1970–1971

In August 1970, as there were no further developments with the Hammersmith post, Olga, Jaroslav and I prepared to fly to Boston so that I could start the research job at the Children's Hospital there. My one recollection of the flight out was that at the age of thirty-six I finally got a chance to taste a Manhattan. It was delicious. The cocktail was a combination of bourbon, sweet vermouth, Angostura bitters and a cocktail cherry. Our first impression of the USA on this occasion was less favourable. Late in the evening at Logan Airport we spotted a pair of policemen armed with pistols and wearing bulletproof vests. Dressed in black uniforms, they reminded Olga and me of the German Gestapo.

A friend of ours had arranged accommodation, but it would not be ready for three weeks. Fortunately a new colleague of mine from Boston, Walter Gamble, of the famous Proctor and Gamble family, had invited us to stay in his home on Longwood Avenue, about five minutes' walk from the hospital. He said that we would be doing him a favour if we made use of one of his automobiles. His family was in the Maine countryside for the summer, and they had a spare car standing idle in the city. We were most grateful for his generosity.

Jaroslav started school in Brookline in Boston with Robbie, the oldest of Walter Gamble's three sons. He loved it, although a month after our arrival he came home and asked if the sweets his fellow students were offering him might be drugs. The next day I went to see the headmaster who checked the situation and found that heroin was indeed on sale at the school.

My job was very different from the busy surgical position I had held in London. I was working in the research laboratory across the road from the hospital. The head there was Grier Monro, while the second-in-command was Walter Gamble. Our project was to experiment on the long-term preservation of a dog's heart. The work was being conducted because the care of a human heart before transplantation is so crucial. It was important research, but it could be tedious, especially when I had to 'babysit' a heart overnight. In addition to my lab activities I worked at an adolescent cardiology clinic once a week run by Stella Van Praagh, the wife of Richard Van Praagh, a famous pathologist. The clinic offered good experience, and I had some expertise to contribute. At that time Dr Gross, an undisputed hero of paediatric cardiac surgery and head of the department at the Children's Hospital for many years, was nearing retirement, and the standard of heart surgery there was in decline. At the end of the clinic we joined Stella and discussed the patients we had seen. Often I would suggest surgical treatment, but the response was frequently ambivalent. 'We can't do it here. The patient won't survive, and as we have already sent one patient to Birmingham and two to the Mayo Clinic this month we can't send any more. We'll have to wait.' This sort of thing was frustrating, but in general I enjoyed my work.

We spent a weekend with the Gamble family in their summer cottage in Maine. Apart from being almost eaten alive by mosquitoes, it was a wonderful introduction to New England's wilderness. And in winter there were great opportunities to go skating in Boston. Olga spent a considerable amount of time in the excellent medical library there. It was, however, her first experience of American air-conditioning, and she sat with two sweaters on even in high summer. Meanwhile we were somewhat bewildered by the advice we received on driving around the city. We were told if we got lost never to stop and ask for directions, particularly not in downtown Boston, as it was considered too dangerous. Instead, we were advised to keep going until we saw road signs that would help us find our way to our destination. It was not like Czechoslovakia or Britain.

About three months after our arrival I received a letter from London. Iain Aberdeen, by now a good friend, had decided to emigrate to Philadelphia after toying with the idea for over a year. He felt that to make one's mark in cardiac surgery one had to work in the USA. Although all his friends, including myself, tried to persuade him not to transfer he was adamant. He had always maintained that paediatric cardiac surgery was very much a team effort, but when he decided to cross the Atlantic he seemed to have forgotten this and took with him no professional support; no assistant, nurse or perfusionist. He was replacing John Waldhausen, a fast and technically excellent surgeon. Moreover the diagnostic accuracy at Great Ormond Street Hospital was far superior to that of the hospital in Philadelphia. Bill Rashkind in Philadelphia was a great researcher; his development of balloon or Rashkind septostomy was a milestone in paediatric cardiology, but for routine investigations he was no match for Mike Tynan, Ian Carr or Gerald Graham at Great Ormond Street. Iain Aberdeen was a great organizer but a very slow surgeon. The consistently excellent results achieved in London were very much down to David Waterston and to the outstanding calibre of the senior registrars who handled post-operative care. In the event, it proved a bad move for Iain.

I had a few letters from Great Ormond Street from former colleagues saying that they would like me to return and take over his job, but then a missive arrived from Richard Bonham Carter, known as Dick, a senior cardiologist at the hospital. He said that although he would very much like me to rejoin the team there was very little chance of my getting the job. The last eight consultant appointments in cardiac surgery in the UK had gone to foreigners, and the opinion in the country was that it was time for this trend to stop. But I was not prepared to give up that easily.

I decided to fly back and talk to those involved in person. The next day Olga drove me to Logan Airport, and I went off to buy a plane ticket. I presented a cheque, but the clerk required a credit card. I explained that I had been in Boston only for three months and didn't have one. He asked if I had any substantial debt, and I assured him that I had never been in debt. Surprisingly, this didn't go down well. 'Without a debit or credit card or a debt as a guarantee I can't sell you a ticket.' I suggested that he contact my boss, Professor Nadas from the Children's Hospital, who could vouch for me. 'You're a doctor?' he enquired. When I confirmed this he said, 'Well, I may need you one day – so here's your ticket.'

I flew to London and visited Dick Bonham Carter at his home. He was kind and supportive but restated that he thought my chances of getting the job were slim. Next day David Waterston invited me to dinner. In his usual laconic manner he said, 'Don't worry, Jarda. Come for the interview. I think you have a good chance.' So I duly sent in my application.

The next three weeks was spent in Boston rehearsing my interview with Olga. All medical jobs in Czechoslovakia were decided on the basis of a written application and references, and there was no face-to-face interview.

My only previous experience of one had been at Hammersmith Hospital, so I tried to go through all the possible permutations of questions with Olga. Back at Great Ormond Street on the day I was delighted to discover that I was prepared for every topic raised. Afterwards they asked all the candidates to wait in a room together, and the one whose name was called out had got the job. So I had a tense forty minutes sitting with two former colleagues and friends who had worked with me at Great Ormond Street: Phil Deverall and Chris Lincoln. They enquired whether I had been asked any stupid questions during my interview such as the role of the psychologist in paediatric cardiac surgery. This had not seemed especially tricky to me, as Olga and I had prepared an answer for this, but I remained apprehensive. When my name was called I was in seventh heaven! After the interview, driving back in the dark to Blackheath where I was staying with a friend, I was so jubilant that I found myself on the wrong side of the road with car lights coming straight at me. I quickly swerved back across the central line.

I cut short my year's research in the USA, as Iain Aberdeen left Great Ormond Street on 1 January. They appointed an American senior registrar, Keith Ashcraft, as my locum and gave me three months to complete my research in Boston. Before leaving to return to London in March 1971 I made a brief trip to the Mayo Clinic and got a chance to visit Pittsburgh and Baltimore. Dwight McGoon, the senior cardiac surgeon at the clinic, was incredibly kind. Every morning he collected me in his car from my motel, drove me to the clinic and made sure I saw as much as possible. I was extremely impressed by the standard of surgery and the organization of the clinic for both in-patients and out-patients.

During the last week I went to Birmingham, Alabama, to meet the senior cardiac surgeon, John Kirklin, there. I was somewhat apprehensive about this, as I had got the Great Ormond Street job over Phil Deverall, who had a strong supporter in Dr Kirklin. Phil had worked in Birmingham as a fellow for a year, and Kirklin had formed a very high opinion of him.

In fact, Dr Kirklin was away when I arrived and was due to return the following day. He had two visitors to his surgery at that time: Dr Lieberman, a cardiac surgeon from Tel Aviv, and me. His secretary gave us a message from her boss that we should come to the theatre the next day but only one of us for each operation.

I chose the second case, a Mustard operation on a nine-month-old child who had previously had a Blalock–Hanlon atrial septectomy. The atmosphere in the theatre was very tense, with nobody saying a word. I stood next to the anaesthetist and watched the operation. After about thirty minutes Dr Kirklin turned to me and said, 'Dr Stark, are we doing it correctly?' I found this hard to answer. At the time Great Ormond Street had the best results for transposition operations, but you do not tell the god of cardiac surgery that he might be doing something wrong. Late that afternoon Dr Kirklin took me to the university club for a drink, after which we stopped at the hospital to examine the child and then he dropped me off at my hotel.

In the morning he returned to collect me at 6.45. We went straight to the intensive care unit. The child was somewhat dusky in colour and his breathing rather laboured. Dr Kirklin explained to me that they did not ventilate patients post-operatively but used the Gregory Technique: constant positive airway pressure or CPAP. It was a relatively new technique, and in London we did not have much experience with it except when weaning patients off a ventilator.

At any rate, soon after we arrived in the unit the technicians started to measure the child's cardiac output using the dye dilution technique. But as soon as they injected the dye the patient went into ventricular tachycardia, then fibrillation, arrested and died. It was profoundly upsetting.

Dr Kirklin in his usual methodical manner asked for a post mortem and called a conference that afternoon. During this he asked me if I had spotted any mistakes in post-operative care. I had noticed that the patient had continued to bleed during the night – not a massive amount but a steady blood loss. When I calculated the quantity I realized that the child had lost two and a half times his blood volume. Moreover after all the transfusions his pH was quite alkalotic. I had mentioned this, but Dr Kirklin confidently assured us that the departmental criteria for reopening the child owing to bleeding had not been breached. They had protocols for everything, but the problem was that their criteria were extrapolated from adult patients. When I pointed this out Dr Kirklin asked if I could write down the Great Ormond Street criteria for reopening after bleeding, and he implemented these for his own department's protocol with immediate effect. This I found very impressive.

Another test came the next day when I joined the ward round. In the second room Dr Kirklin sat in the chair at the bedside of a patient, handed the stethoscope to his other visitor and said, 'Dr Lieberman, listen and give me your diagnosis.' The Israeli surgeon pronounced that the patient, a 23-year-old male, had an aortic incompetence. Then it was my turn to give my opinion. I was never very good at auscultating heart murmurs because of my poor musical ear, so I was unsure what to say. It did not sound like a simple aortic incompetence to me. I wondered whether to repeat the experienced adult cardiac surgeon's diagnosis or stick my neck out. I decided on the latter and said that I thought the patient had a ventricular septal defect or VSD with aortic incompetence. Dr Kirklin looked at me for what seemed ages. Finally he confirmed that the patient had a VSD, had developed endocarditis and that part of his aortic leaflet had been destroyed, causing severe aortic incompetence.

After this I could do no wrong. On all subsequent visits to Birmingham I was invited to stay at Dr Kirklin's house, going with him daily to the hospital. He was always 100 per cent supportive and said I could call him any time for advice. Later he wrote me a very cordial letter asking if his junior colleague, Al Pacifico, could visit our department at Great Ormond Street to learn about transposition surgery and added that he would like to join him for the last few days. I felt really honoured.

13
BACK IN LONDON, EARLY 1970S

After returning from the USA to London in spring 1971 I started as a consultant. I really enjoyed it, but it was hard work, as I spent ten to twelve hours in the hospital each day. In addition to that, I was on call every other day and every other weekend. My colleague and former mentor David Waterston was close to retirement, so I covered most of his 'on calls' as well. At that point we were living in Clare Court in one of the hospital flats near by. The day we moved in Jaroslav, aged eleven, went to the shops on his own initiative and bought a five-litre can of disinfectant. The flat was filthy; it was hard to imagine that the previous occupants had been doctors. It was also damp, so when one spilled coffee powder on the floor a pool of coffee formed. Jaroslav started school near Parliament Hill Fields and seemed very happy there. About three weeks later he came home and told his mother, 'Oli, I think you should just speak Czech, which you're very good at. Your English is terrible!'

We started looking for a house to buy. Olga thought that perhaps a flat would suit us better, as we were accustomed to living in apartments back in Czechoslovakia, but my preference was to have a house with a garden, and anyway good flats were relatively more expensive than houses in those days. We found a promising-looking one near Parliament Hill Fields, an area we knew as we played tennis there regularly. However, it was too pricey. One could get a mortgage up to three times one's annual salary, and my starting salary as a consultant was £5,500 per year, so we could not afford Hampstead prices.

But then we got lucky. One weekend we visited our Czech friends Jiří and Nina Trnka who lived in Blackheath and with whom we played tennis. While Olga was playing a match with Nina I was reading the *Sunday Times* and came across an advertisement for a house in Anson Road in north London.

BACK IN LONDON, EARLY 1970S

It seemed perfect and was a fair price, but as it was already mid-morning I assumed it had probably been snapped up. I phoned to check and discovered that it was still available. We went to view it on Monday, and we made an offer. It has remained my London home ever since.

The previous owner had strange taste. He had painted all the window frames on the first floor shocking-pink. He had also built a rickety garden shed, which was so awful that one of the first things we did was demolish it. Olga started decorating the upstairs rooms using a handbook on home decoration, a 'how-to' guide that had to be translated for the most part by Jaroslav. For the downstairs two living-rooms we felt we should call in professional help. The two decorators started work, and on the second day Olga asked the men to come upstairs, saying, 'Why do you think we asked you to do this work?' They were perplexed. The reason was simple, she continued. 'We thought that you'd do a better job than I'm doing up here. But, quite frankly, I don't think you are.' The senior decorator didn't blink but asked if he could use the phone and called his boss. 'George, the lady is fussy. She wants a proper job.' And then he turned to Olga and said, 'Mum, it'll be ten quid more. Is that OK?' Olga and I thought: That's British workmen for you!

My own job was very satisfying. The team at Great Ormond Street started to operate on smaller and smaller babies with greatly improved results. As the hospital was renowned for its child heart surgery all over the world I was invited to lecture abroad. Moreover I did not have to work hard to build up my private practice as it was such a well-established department and there were very few in Europe operating on infants with congenital heart defects. Within a short time my waiting list for private patients, 99 per cent of whom came from abroad, was eighteen months. As I was not keen to operate at weekends I was happy to refer some of the patients to my consultant colleague. This struck some as unusual and unorthodox, as they felt that cardiologists would not continue to refer patients to me.

We performed an excellent series of Mustard operations for transposition of the great arteries during the first year of life, and I submitted a paper to the American Association for Thoracic Surgery (AATS) which was holding a major meeting in Las Vegas. I had no doubt that it would be accepted, so I booked the flights and the hotel in advance. One reason I was keen to attend was the fact that I had always wanted to see the Grand Canyon. I was amazed when the paper was turned down, as we had performed Mustard operations on fifty-two babies with just two deaths. When I arrived at the meeting I realized what lay behind the rejection. There was another paper being presented on the same subject, except that the numbers were smaller – that is, eight babies with four deaths – and it was being presented by a member of the programme committee. I had prepared a slide for the discussion afterwards, complimenting the authors on their results and showing ours for comparison, indicating that we had perhaps used a slightly different approach. Many attendees came up to congratulate me at the end of the session.

Professor Alexander Nadas from Boston suggested during the meeting that we should play the fruit machines in one of the main casinos. He played quarters, while I played nickels. After fifteen minutes I hit the jackpot and had four plastic coffee cups full of nickels. Of course my winnings had evaporated within half an hour or so, as the machines are set up so that the casino never loses. Another day my friend Dino Tatooles took me to MGM, the largest casino in Las Vegas. Before we went in he placed several $100 bills in my old attaché case in such a way that they were partially sticking out. As the case was anyway quite bulgy it appeared as if it was crammed with a lot of banknotes. He suggested I amble slowly down the central aisle. I created a sensation. Everybody stopped playing and had their eyes glued on me. The effect was immediate and very gratifying.

As predicted, the highlight of my trip was undoubtedly a visit to the Grand Canyon. I flew to the South Rim, but as it was already relatively late I tried to get a bed in the ranch by the river at the bottom so that I could return early the next day. But the man at the travel agency told me that the ranch was full. Remembering how things worked in Communist Czechoslovakia, I tried my luck by giving him an envelope containing $20 and saying that I would return an hour later to see if there had been a cancellation. And there was!

I immediately started my downward trek of around 18 kilometres. It was wonderful; a fantastic landscape with no hamburger or Coca-Cola stands in sight, just wooden orientation boards with information on geology and wildlife. But by the time I was near the river I felt considerable pain in my heels, so when I reached the bank I sat down and took my walking boots off. There was a large haemorrhagic blister on each heel, as boot nails had worked their way through the sole. I had worn the boots in London for a couple of long walks, but this trek was evidently in a different category. I found myself wondering how I would get to the top the next day. That evening at the ranch was highly enjoyable. A group of geology students from the University of Utah was in residence, and we sat around the campfire and chatted until late. The next day's climb with the blisters on my feet was painful but manageable, the spectacular scenery compensating for my discomfort. Overall it had been a very successful meeting.

Just before a Medical Committee meeting at Great Ormond Street I was approached by the hospital's House Governor who asked me if I wanted to be called Dr or Mr. Then the chairman of the committee, Mr David Mathews, a plastic surgeon, came up to ask the same question. In the UK all surgeons who pass the Fellowship of the Royal College of Surgeons examination are called Mr. If the doctor in question is female she would be called Miss, irrespective of whether she was single or married. I told them that it should be the hospital's decision. As I did not have a fellowship (FRCS) I should more correctly be called Dr, but perhaps for the referring physicians it would be confusing and it might be better if I was called Mr. When the matter came up for discussion, as was customary I left the room. When I returned I discovered that they couldn't agree, as both the house governor and Mr Mathews reported differently my answer to their question, so a special Medical Committee meeting had to be convened to resolve this issue. They eventually concluded that I should be called Mr.

I felt that perhaps I should make the effort to sit the FRCS examination. I was not especially keen, because it was notoriously difficult. Many of the Great Ormond Street surgeons had failed it at least once. And by then I was thirteen years post-graduation, so my knowledge of the basic sciences was vanishing fast. I wrote to the Royal College and sent its administrators my curriculum vitae. They replied that I was six months short on training in A&E and would have to spend six months in an A&E department, and then I could reapply for the fellowship. In a way, I was relieved, because this was unworkable. Great Ormond Street had appointed me as a consultant cardiothoracic surgeon, and my colleagues would not be keen for me to go off to work elsewhere for six months. At any rate the situation was resolved in 1980 when the Royal College awarded me an honorary FRCS.

Life in London was hectic but enjoyable. Jaroslav's teacher at primary school, Mr Riddler, had suggested that he apply for Westminster Public School and also for William Ellis School, a state school with an excellent reputation. As the latter was about fifteen minutes' walk from our home we decided he should apply there rather than Westminster. The headmaster asked us as parents to sit through the interview but not to interfere. So we sat quietly in the corner and followed the proceedings. The headmaster said, 'Jaroslav, you started school in Czechoslovakia, then emigrated to England, then went to Boston and now you're back in England. Have you not found the changes disruptive?' Our eleven-year-old had a quick answer. 'Not really, sir. Being exposed to different educational systems was probably beneficial to me.' The headmaster had difficulty keeping a straight face.

William Ellis was very good for Jaroslav. His mathematics teacher soon recognized his aptitude for the subject, so he suggested that our son did not attend classes. Instead he gave him books to read on his own, and as a consequence Jaroslav was doing calculus about three years before his class caught up. When he was sixteen we arranged a ten-week French course in Nice for him. We had been somewhat concerned that when he was younger we had dragged him through too many museums, galleries and cathedrals and that we might have put him off art and history for good. But while he was in Nice he sent us postcards from the Musée Chagall, the Musée Matisse, the Fondation Maeght and others. We were delighted. He was a very good student, so when the time came for him to make a decision about which subjects to take for his A levels all his teachers wanted him to do their subject. Olga was firm. 'You are good at maths, so you will take maths and special maths, physics and special physics.' He hardly worked at all for his A levels, yet he got four A-plus results and a scholarship to Cambridge.

Before Jaroslav went to university he dated Isy, a lovely girl a year his junior. I remember the horror with which my parents greeted the news after I sent them a photograph of the couple. Isy was black; her parents came from Trinidad. People with black skin were almost never seen in Prague, and there was a great deal of prejudice. Olga and I kept in touch with her long after the teenagers stopped seeing one another. By then Isy had a child, but her boyfriend did not want to marry her, so Olga and I supported her through her medical studies.

While in Cambridge Jaroslav started going out with Lucy, a girl with a very strong personality. In the summer they planned to go on holiday in

BACK IN LONDON, EARLY 1970S

Greece and Italy. They were four couples, but at the last minute the three other boys pulled out, so Jaroslav went alone with all four girls. It was quite entertaining. The girls had made arrangements that one of them would call home once a week; then the parents concerned would inform the others. So we were getting calls from the parents of the girls on a regular basis. 'All is well. Your boy is still looking after the girls.'

When Jaroslav split up with Lucy he was devastated. But then he met Sandra. Olga and I were skiing over Christmas in Verbier in Switzerland one year, while he was with the Skiing Club of Great Britain in Tignes. It had snowed heavily for a few days in the Savoi Alps, and Jaroslav and his associates had spent most of their time huddled up in bed. When he came to join us in Verbier he was carrying an extra pair of skis. Olga and I were somewhat taken aback as Jaroslav generally liked to travel light. Apparently, a doctor who had been skiing in Tignes was travelling to a conference, so Jaroslav was helping out. We did not comprehend immediately that the doctor was his new girlfriend Sandra, who had two degrees and a Ph.D.

They got on well, and she was very good for him, as she was a no-nonsense girl. When he got a first in one of his Cambridge examinations she did not feel that it was good enough, as she thought he was capable of honours. A minor problem was that she was some twelve years older than he. At parties Sandra's friends mistook Jaroslav for her son, and in the company of his friends she could seem more of a mother figure than a girlfriend. Sandra came to realize this and eventually terminated the relationship.

Later on in Cambridge he met Kate. She was a year his junior and already engaged to someone else – although ultimately this didn't seem to present a problem to the blossoming of their relationship. One summer they went on holiday together to Corfu. When they came back they timidly showed us the engagement rings they had bought there. I think it was the best thing that could have happened to them both.

Jaroslav and Kate had an excellent marriage. In addition, they worked together professionally remarkably well. Kate was a researcher in *in vitro* fertilization at London's Hammersmith Hospital, based in Robert Winston's department. She would perform experiments, and Jaroslav would undertake statistical and mathematical evaluation and modelling. One year their paper was accepted at a large international meeting of obstetricians. A few days beforehand Kate caught a bad cold, so Jaroslav presented the paper and handled the discussion. I think their professional cooperation gave him the idea of establishing the Centre for Integrative Systems Biology and Bioinformatics (CISBIO), of which he became a director. The postgraduate students there had two supervisors, a biologist or doctor and a mathematician. Later when he moved to Imperial College he established his institute there, which was also very successful.

Unfortunately Kate had problems with her parents, for soon after she wed Jaroslav they told her that she had married beneath her – as Jaroslav was a 'foreigner'. The fact that he was a professor at University College London and editor of the most prestigious mathematics journal in the country made no difference. One year we went on holiday to northern Corsica and took her younger sister Rosie with us. During the vacation we noticed a small lump on the side of her neck. We insisted that after her return to London she should be seen urgently by specialists. Hodgkin's lymphoma was diagnosed. It was agreed that she should undergo treatment at Hammersmith Hospital where Kate was working. It took around six months, during which time Rosie stayed with Jaroslav and Kate. The treatment was successful, and the last time she was seen as an out-patient her father Peter accompanied her. He asked for copies of all the medical reports. As they were not immediately available the doctors told him that they would prepare them within the next two days and give them to Kate to forward to him. Peter duly left with Rosie, but that evening he telephoned Kate. Speaking, it seemed, completely irrationally, he told her that her and her husband's behaviour towards Rosie was completely unacceptable and therefore he and his wife did not want to have anything more to do with them. That was that. As a result they never came to see Daniel, their only grandson at the time.

Soon after my appointment at Great Ormond Street I started to receive invitations to meetings and conferences abroad because our thoracic unit was internationally renowned. Early on I visited departments in Montreal, Pittsburgh and Durham (Duke University) and attended an American Association for Cardiology meeting in Anaheim. I was also visiting professor in Los Angeles and San Francisco.

About six months after starting as a consultant at Great Ormond Street I had a phone call from Glen Rosenquist, an American cardiologist who had spent six months of his sabbatical at our hospital. By this time he was chairman of paediatrics at the University of Omaha in Nebraska. He told me that his department was looking for a new head of paediatric cardiac surgery. He knew that I was shortly travelling to the USA to present a paper at a meeting of American Heart Association and wondered if I might stop in Omaha to discuss the appointment with them. I had been very friendly with Glen while he was in London, so I agreed to this. The department duly sent me a ticket and booked me into a hotel near the university.

When I arrived I found a schedule for the next two days in my room. I immediately realized that I was to be interviewed as a candidate for the job – not as an adviser, as I had presumed. It was late afternoon, so I had time to consider my position. I decided to call Dr John Kirklin, the most respected cardiac surgeon in the world who was by now a very good friend. I explained the situation, pointing out that I was really not interested in the job but for the sake of the interview would need to know the main negotiating points. He said it was simple. There was just one important issue: I should be able to keep control of all the money I made, as I would have to buy equipment, hire nurses and so on.

Armed with his advice I went to breakfast with the chancellor. He was very pleasant and filled me in on the medical school and the university in general. My next appointment was with the dean of the Medical School. He got straight to the point. 'Your salary will be $200,000 and on top of that there is quite a big private practice.' (My salary in London at that time was £5,500, the equivalent of $13,000.) He continued, 'Out of that you will keep 20 per cent, 20 per cent will go to your division, 20 per cent to the Department of Cardiac Surgery, 20 per cent to the Department of Surgery and 20 per cent to the Medical School. What do you think?' Bearing in mind what John Kirklin had told me, I said that it did not sound right to me. So what did I have in mind, the Dean asked. I replied that 20 per cent going to me was fine, but 60 per cent should go straight to my division; the rest they could distribute as they wished. He agreed to this immediately.

This demonstrated to me that in the USA if a hospital really wanted to hire someone the sky was the limit regarding salary. I thanked the dean and said I would discuss it with my wife and let the medical school know my decision within the next two weeks. After my return to London Olga and I spent several hours trying to compose a suitably polite letter saying that I did not want to swap London for Omaha, Nebraska, at that stage of my career.

Then an invitation came from George Stalpaert, chief of cardiac surgery in Leuven, Belgium. He invited me to give two lectures and to show his staff how we performed a Mustard operation for transposition of the great arteries. I went with Helmuth Oelert from Hanover, our senior registrar, who was to assist me. When we arrived George took us from the airport to our hotel, and a couple of hours later he brought us to his house where we had a wonderful evening meal. At about 11.30 I suggested it was time to go to bed, as we had surgery the following morning. George responded that we would not be operating that day, as it was a Belgian national holiday. So we opened another bottle of delicious red wine.

Consequently I was taken by surprise at 2.30 a.m. when, with a straight face, he told us we were due in surgery at 8.30 that morning. There was, in fact, no national holiday. I thought this outrageous. We returned to our hotel, and I told George I wanted to examine the data and talk to the parents of the child before operating, which meant him driving us into his department in good time. But he had to take several of his children to school first, so he didn't arrive to collect us from the hotel until 9.15, and I was increasingly annoyed. In the hospital there was no sign of the parents, and he told me that the chest of the child had already been opened. By then I was furious. We went to theatre, and I performed the Mustard operation with his assistance.

The problem was that their perfusionists were not accustomed to handling small children, therefore terminating the perfusion was difficult. When I asked them to reduce the flow, the venous pressure dropped so much so that I was worried about getting air into the heart. When I asked them to increase the venous pressure, the heart overfilled to bursting point. I finally resolved the problem by coming off bypass at a low venous pressure and transfusing the patient with small increments of 25 ml of blood. This worked.

The next day they scheduled another Mustard, and it went more smoothly. I told George that I would assist him with a third child. He did not comment on this, but the theatre nurses later came over and pleaded with me not to let the professor operate. I insisted, because I felt they had to learn the correct procedure. What I did not realize was what a test this third operation would be on my nerves. Clearly the surgeons and nurses had no experience with children, so even the cannulation of the superior vena cava and inferior vena cava was a major problem. Some time later George sent

Wim Daenen, his assistant, to us as a senior registrar, and Wim became a successful congenital heart surgeon in subsequent years.

In 1972 David Waterston was invited to a meeting of the German and Austrian General Paediatric Surgeons in Obergurgl, Austria. This was an excellent skiing resort, and the meeting was organized around this activity. A few days beforehand David fell ill and asked me to attend in his place and to present his paper on colon replacement of the oesophagus, his signature operation. I arrived late in the afternoon not knowing anyone.

In the evening I went to the bar, and while having a drink I overheard a conversation between a pair of elderly surgeons sitting adjacent to my table. The two men were speaking in German of my friends David Waterston and Iain Aberdeen in not especially genial terms. I kept quiet, but the following morning my lecture was the first of the day. I went to the podium and explained in German that David Waterston was ill and that I would present his talk. As he had prepared it with English-language slides I said I would speak in English but assured them that I would be happy to handle the subsequent discussion in German. The two men from the previous night were sitting in the first row, clearly distinguished professors. I could see that they recognized me from the bar, and it dawned on them that I had understood their conversation the previous evening. Their faces went ashen. I think they were really embarrassed. I thought: Fifteen–love.

In May 1972 I was invited to Bergen to give a lecture on the surgical treatment of ventricular septal defect in infancy. We had a long-standing arrangement with Bergen Hospital. Its cardiologists would investigate the young patients there and then send them over to us in London. A Norwegian patient would be flown in with a doctor and a nurse, while some emergency cases were intubated, ventilated and put on a intravenous drip. They also brought two or three units of cross-matched blood with the infant. Patients often arrived in a better condition than ones living less than 80 kilometres from London. We could operate within a few hours, so we had a very satisfactory working relationship.

Later that year I went to a meeting of the European Society of Paediatric Cardiologists in Uppsala to present a paper on post-operative care in infant cardiac surgery. They took us to the city's museum to see the famous Silver Bible but were none too pleased when I told them that the Swedish Army had stolen the Bible from Prague during the Thirty Years War.

14
LONDON, 1973–1974

Not long after I had been appointed to the consultant post at Great Ormond Street I had a call from a secretary from the Czech Embassy. She asked me if I could help with a Czech child with a very complex congenital heart defect. I said of course, as we operated on children from all over the world. Then I added, tongue in cheek, that if they were sending such a child to the West it was highly likely that he or she was the son or daughter of a prominent politician; in such cases it was unusual for such patients to be operated on by a criminal. The secretary was bewildered. I had to explain. I had been sentenced to a year in a labour camp for leaving the country at the time I did, therefore I was a criminal. However, I pointed out, the Czech constitution was clear that anyone who desired could leave the country without such a penalty. The secretary said that she would have to consult her ambassador and phone me back. Ten minutes later she called again. 'The Ambassador says it's OK.' This was typical. When senior Czech politicians needed a favour from you, things could be smoothed out, but not the other way round. My parents and my sister were not allowed to visit me in the UK for a number of years.

Olga and I were meanwhile leading very busy lives. She moved from doing research in microbiology to working in paediatrics under Professor Otto Wolff, and she was running an obesity clinic. The Professor believed that the best way to treat obese children was to hospitalize them for six weeks on a regime of 800 calories a day. Olga was not convinced by this practice and discussed it with a number of experts in the UK and abroad, and she came to the conclusion that the regime was pointless. Once the children were discharged they reverted to their usual eating habits and put the weight back on in no time. We were interested to note that when Professor Wolff retired, his successor, Professor – later Dame – June Lloyd, agreed with Olga, and the department ended the practice at Great Ormond Street.

One patient who attended the clinic was Jeremy, an obese child of wealthy lawyer parents. On a previous visit Olga had given them a diet sheet and told them that their son should lose about eight pounds in around six weeks. When they came back they were clearly unhappy. They told Olga that Jeremy had not lost any weight. She explained that the only explanation was that Jeremy had not adhered to the diet. They were indignant. 'He followed the diet exactly as prescribed,' they said. She asked if she could speak with the boy on his own. They left the room, and he admitted that every evening he set his alarm clock for two in the morning when he would sneak into the kitchen and eat a large bowl of cereal topped up with full-fat milk or cream. This explained his lack of progress in losing weight.

Olga and I liked to have lunch together at Mille Pini, an Italian restaurant next to St George's Church on the corner of Queen Square, where they served good food and where there was a convivial atmosphere. One day we walked in and all the tables were occupied apart from one. It was a table for four, and a man was sitting alone. We guessed he was from the law courts near by, as he wore a pin-striped suit and looking highly distinguished. We asked if we could join him, and he said that was fine. Olga and I proceeded to chat together in a combination of English and Czech. Our companion at the table suddenly asked in perfect Czech where we were from. Olga and I were stunned – and frantically tried to recall whether we had used any swearwords when we thought no one could understand us. It turned out that he was married to a young Czech woman. He had met her after the war when he was a RAF officer in Prague. To our further surprise we discovered that his wife was a close relative of our friend Vojta Volavka. It was a small world.

In 1973 I was invited to the Hospital La Paz in Madrid. Paco Alvarez was in charge, and Pedro Sanchez, a good friend of mine, worked there. At 5 p.m. they drove me from the airport to my hotel, promising to take me out for dinner at 10.30 that evening. It was my first introduction to Spanish late-night culture, and by the time they collected me I was pretty hungry. In the event, the meal was delicious; it was the first time I had tasted baby eels, which the Spaniards cooked by throwing them live into boiling oil.

That year I also visited Boston's Children's Hospital, acted as a visiting professor at the University of Miami, lectured in Valencia and took part in a meeting of the European Cardiac Surgeons' Club in Oslo. The last was a very interesting trip, as I got the chance to visit the superb Munch Museum there.

The World Congress of the International Society of Cardiovascular Surgery was held in Valencia in September 1973. I was one of the invited speakers in the symposium on Infant Cardiac Surgery. My topic was surgery for transposition in the first year of life. Another lecturer was Denton Cooley from the USA, one of the most famous heart surgeons in the world. He was known to have operated on a huge number of patients. My first encounter with him was while still a senior registrar at Great Ormond Street. I had collected data published in a paper called 'Cardiac Surgery in the First Year of Life: Experience with 1,049 Operations'. My colleagues and I had included only groups of infants on whom we performed at least thirty operations. Given Cooley's reputation, I shouldn't have been surprised that a paper from his department was published soon after this entitled 'Experience with 1,050 patients with CHD Operated On During the First Year of Life'. His department had scraped the bottom of the barrel and included even the smallest groups.

During the World Congress Dr Cooley presented a general paper on infant cardiac surgery. When he mentioned transpositions he said that they had tried the Mustard operation on two or three infants but as they all failed to survive they did not operate on infant transpositions any more. When it came to my lecture I was in a quandary. I was to present a series of fifty-two infant Mustards with two deaths. The predicament was how not to offend Dr Cooley and remain tactful. I thought I resolved the problem rather ingeniously. At the beginning of my talk I said that Dr Cooley had presented a lecture on surgery of transposition in relation to historical practice, how such operations had been done a few years earlier, whereas I would present the latest statistics regarding infant heart surgery in London. I then went on to read my paper.

A second issue arose with Dr Brian Barratt-Boyes – later to become Sir Brian Barratt-Boyes – from New Zealand. He presented an excellent paper about the early correction of Fallot's tetralogy with the remarkable results he had achieved. As an argument for early correction he quoted a paper from Great Ormond Street about the results for shunts (palliation). As I had written this I felt the need to comment. I complimented him on his amazing results but pointed out that my paper was about the results for shunts for various complex cyanotic heart conditions, not just for tetralogy. Therefore his argument, using our paper as an example of bad results of shunts compared with his excellent ones for correction, was invalid. His response stunned me. 'You're lying!' he declared.

I was floored by this and kept quiet. Jim Malm from New York was sitting next to me. I knew him well, as we often played tennis at the American meetings. He said, 'Don't worry, Jarda. We'll get the bastard!' Jim's lecture was after the break. Barratt-Boyes presented his results of infant heart surgery conducted under deep hypothermia and circulatory arrest, and Jim followed with the same topic, except that his operations were done on cardiopulmonary bypass. During his talk he showed a slide of a number of grown-up boys and girls, saying that most of his patients operated on bypass were now in college, while most of those operated in deep hypothermia by Barratt-Boyes were probably still in primary school. This implied that patients operated under deep hypothermia were more likely to develop neurological damage. It was also retaliation for Barratt-Boyes's attack on me.

The same year I became a member of the European Cardiac Surgeons' Club. It was very select, with just two members from each European country. They were chosen partly on merit but also on whether they would get on well, listen to one another and not pontificate. So, for example, Sweden was represented not by Viking Björk but Dr Johansson from Uppsala. Iain Aberdeen and Jean-Paul Binet from Paris had started the club, and I was replacing Iain, who by then had moved to Philadelphia, although he continued to attend the meetings for a few years. Ethicon sponsored the club, and Uli Karsten from Hamburg was a great supporter. The meetings took place one Saturday a year. We would arrive on Friday evening, have dinner and decide on the programme for the next day. Saturday was the main meeting day, to be followed by a convivial dinner. Then on Sunday after breakfast we would leave. The local organizer would select a secluded venue, such as a château, a good hotel or similar. Ethicon picked up the tab. Uli was an amazing man who became a good friend to all of us. He never pushed Ethicon products, and eventually we elected him as an honorary member. As it was a small group discussions were very free, and over the years I learned a great deal. Donald Ross and myself were the UK members. From France came Binet and Fontan, from Germany Sebening and Borst, from Holland Jan Nauta, from Norway Gudmund Semb, from Sweden Johansson from Upsala, from Belgium Chalant from Leuven and from Switzerland Charlie Hahn. We had a number of excellent meetings in Oslo, Rotterdam,

Stockholm, Grimonster Castle in Belgium, Malmö, Toledo, Lake Como, Düsseldorf, Hanover, Crans Montana and elsewhere. We were each encouraged to invite a guest to each meeting. One year I invited Bohouš Hučín from Prague. He was running a very good unit and enjoyed the meeting very much.

Not long after I attended a meeting of European Paediatric Cardiologists in London where I presented a paper on 'Obstruction of Venous Return after the Mustard Operation' and took part in a Journée de Travail sur les Malpositions des Gros Vaisseaux in Marseilles.

In 1974 I was invited to give a lecture at the Mayo Clinic and attended the American Association for Thoracic Surgery (AATS) meeting in Las Vegas. That year David Waterston retired, and Marc de Leval applied for his post. He was by far the best candidate. He came from Liège in Belgium and had trained for two years with Frank Gerbode in San Francisco. He then came as a senior registrar to us for a year, before winning a prestigious Evarts E. Graham fellowship from the AATS. He decided to spend it at the Mayo Clinic with Dr Dwight McGoon, one of the giants of cardiac surgery who was not only an excellent surgeon but a lovely man. It was a tragedy when Dwight later developed severe Parkinson's disease.

Marc competed against Ralph Sapsford, a South African who was a reasonable surgeon but not in Marc's class. The other candidate was Brian Pickering, a less able surgeon. At the appointment committee it was crystal-clear who was the best candidate and who should be appointed. However, Bill Cleland, an Australian consultant surgeon at the Hammersmith Hospital, said that we should not appoint another foreigner, suggesting that one – namely myself – was enough. He proposed that we should appoint Marc as a locum consultant for a year, train a British candidate up during this time and then dismiss Marc. I felt this was outrageous and said so. I had the regulations of the Royal College of Surgeons at my fingertips, but it was Audrey Callaghan, wife of the then prime minister Jim Callaghan and chairwoman of the appointments committee, who most effectively opposed the plan. She put her weight firmly behind Marc, saying that the function of the committee was to appoint the best candidate and he was clearly that. We won the day, and Marc became my colleague for the next thirty years. That was fortunate for Great Ormond Street – and especially for me. At one point people said we were the only two cardiac surgeons in the UK working in the same department on speaking terms with one another. Perhaps even more importantly, later on we were the only two surgeons in a single department to be honorary members of the AATS and, even more remarkably, the only two cardiac surgeons to hold an A-plus award from the Department of Health and Social Security.

I was asked to operate on a small Russian baby, Vitali Bakst Lemberg, about eight months old. He was helped to get to the UK by Robert and Evelyn Lyons, whom I later knew as members of Highgate Golf Club. The boy arrived with his mother and was admitted to Great Ormond Street. Investigations showed that he suffered from transposition of the great arteries; in addition, his heart was rotated and twisted so that it was in a highly abnormal position. When I opened his chest my assistant, Ralph Sapsford, said, 'Don't bother. Just make an atrial septal defect as a palliative procedure. Nothing else can be done.' However, I had decided that we must try to save him. We turned the heart upside down, rotated it and operated behind the heart. The boy survived and did well.

Subsequently his parents divorced, and Vitali emigrated to New York with his father. I heard that he was doing well once or twice in later years from my friends the Lyons. The big surprise came many decades later in 2012 when I received an email from New York. Vitali said he had never had any follow-up examination and wondered whether it was advisable, as he felt fine. If I felt it was a good idea he was happy to come to London. I was intrigued, so I arranged a joint examination with my cardiology colleague Dr Philip Rees. Vitali, however, could not come until 2013, by which time Dr Rees had retired, so I arranged the tests and examination with Dr Fiona Walker at the Heart Hospital. To my delight everything was normal. Two days after the examination I was able to meet Vitali informally at the Lyons' home. It was an emotional reunion. We were delighted to be in touch after so much time had passed; Vitali was married with a lovely daughter.

I was busy at Great Ormond Street but had started operating on private patients at the Harley Street Clinic. At Great Ormond Street we could undertake surgery on only 10 per cent of all patients as private patients. The standard of care for cardiac patients was so good that most patients were treated on the NHS, and I generally talked those who wanted private surgery out of it. Occasionally parents would insist, but usually these were situations resulting from marital disagreement when a mother and father were in the throes of an acrimonious separation or divorce. So the total number of my UK private practice amounted to just four or five British patients; the rest came from abroad. As Great Ormond Street was so widely known and well established I did not have to build up referrals from cardiologists around the world. Patients came to the hospital and later on to me personally. I operated at the Harley Street Clinic half a day a week, which was later expanded to one-and-a-half days a week. As I was not keen to operate electively on Saturdays I referred some of my private patients to Marc de Leval, who proved an excellent surgeon and colleague.

In the UK there were several cardiac clubs reserved for surgeons of a similar age. They used to meet once a year to discuss common problems. The discussions were generally uninhibited. One such organization, Pete's Club, had a single rule for presentations. You could discuss anything you liked, but it must not give you any credit. In other words, presentations of mistakes and failures was the order of the day rather than successful surgery. Soon after I was appointed a consultant in 1971 Professor Bentall from the Hammersmith Hospital approached me to join Pete's Club. He said, 'We're a similar age, so you'll enjoy it.' I was not minded to refuse, even though most of its members were at least ten years older than me. It was certainly a good society, as one could learn a great deal from the mistakes of others.

I recall one meeting where Gerard Brom from Leiden, a doyen of European cardiothoracic surgery, presented an interesting case. During open-heart surgery on a small child, after a period of circulatory arrest he discovered the arterial line and the aorta full of air; this was disastrous, but he found a swift solution. He disconnected the lines and reconnected the arterial line to the venous system and started pumping arterial blood into the patient's venous system – a technique known as reverse circulation. When the patient was full of blood, air bubbles started coming out of the aorta and then blood. As soon as air bubbles stopped coming from the aorta he clamped the lines, then reconnected them in the normal fashion, rewarmed the patient and completed the surgical procedure.

About eight months later I experienced a similar problem. I was operating on a six-month-old baby with a ventricular septal defect. As the venous return was excessive I cooled the patient and introduced a short period of circulatory arrest. I was not sure how the air got into the arterial line, but I suppose the pump was not fully occlusive. The fact that I knew how to handle the situation and did not panic impressed everyone in theatre. Thanks to Gerald Brom and Pete's Club the patient survived and was discharged home a week later.

About a year after the first meeting of Pete's Club that I attended we were having dinner in Hendon Hall. Olga was sitting between Marvin Sturridge, a surgeon from the Middlesex Hospital, and an adult cardiac surgeon from Charing Cross Hospital. I was sitting opposite them on the other side of the table and could hear their conversation. The Charing Cross surgeon was talking across Olga to Marvin. He said he had heard that Great Ormond Street was in trouble because Iain Aberdeen had left and they had appointed a 'nobody' from Eastern Europe. Marvin, who knew me well, was frantically gesticulating, trying to draw his colleague's attention to the fact that the lady sitting between them was that nobody's wife – but in vain. Marvin eventually interrupted, saying, 'I think I have not introduced you to Olga, the wife of the new Great Ormond Street surgeon, Jarda Stark from Czechoslovakia.' At this point I chipped in. Earlier Marvin had been saying how much he enjoyed the range of cardiac surgery with which he was involved, from infants with congenital defects to valve surgery and coronaries in adults. So I told them that I had just spent a week with John Kirklin in Alabama who did not think there was a place any longer for the same surgeons operating on babies as well as adults, as they were two specialist disciplines. Marvin was immediately on the defensive. He said that he operated on children at the Middlesex only when we surgeons at Great Ormond Street could not cope. Given the previously dismissive attitude of the Charing Cross surgeon, I enjoyed the situation greatly.

On the whole, however, UK cardiothoracic surgeons welcomed my presence and were very cordial to me. Only the occasional defensive older surgeon – possibly not an especially competent technician – would be hostile. An example was when I was scheduled to speak at the National Society of Cardiothoracic Surgeons of Great Britain and Ireland and the chairman announced that the next paper would be presented by 'Dr Stark'. This was a classic putdown, since as I had all my surgical qualifications from Czechoslovakia but had not yet been made a Fellow of the Royal College of Surgeons (FRCS).

I started inviting members of the cardiac team from the Kardiocentrum in Prague to our department. At that time my name could not appear on the invitations, which had to be signed by my secretary or one of my colleagues. We organized positions of house surgeons (*sekundář*), senior registrars (assistants) for some, and one, Vaclav Chaloupecky, a cardiologist from Prague, was appointed as a locum consultant *intensivist*. In addition to several young surgeons we had visiting cardiologists and anaesthetists, so that the group could benefit from seeing all London's latest techniques. The Czechs received a full salary and free accommodation at Great Ormond Street, although before leaving Prague most had to sign a declaration that while in Britain they would not contact Czech émigrés. This was nonsense: everyone was aware that they were coming to my department,

Over the years we always had three senior registrars or fellows. One post was reserved for UK trainees; two were for overseas surgeons. Iain Aberdeen, who secured finance from the Department of Health, had initiated the scheme, which attracted excellent candidates from the best US universities, and Marc and I carried on along the same lines. For young surgeons interested in congenital heart surgery it was an attractive post. They had finished their gruelling training in the USA, usually as chief residents, but the number of congenital heart patients they had seen was usually fairly small. To come to Great Ormond Street was a great opportunity. Within a few years people started writing to me when they were entering a cardiac programme, and I would arrange to interview them at one of the US meetings. Very often we had to choose between thirty and forty candidates. Later on another type of candidate emerged. The heads of cardiac surgery departments from European countries would ask us to take one of their most promising young surgeons for training. This was the case with Helmuth Oelert from Hanover, Pavel Horvath from Prague, Pedro Bastos from Porto, Adriano Garotti from Bambino Gesù in Rome and many others. We had to select very carefully, because on the basis of CVs and training alone the Americans were, on paper, considerably better qualified. But we felt responsible for the training of Europeans, and on the whole these individuals were excellent, dedicated young surgeons who contributed greatly to the success of our unit.

The UK senior registrars presented an issue. Great Ormond Street was involved in a cardiac rotation with the Middlesex, Hammersmith and Harefield hospitals. The senior registrars had carried out little or no paediatric cardiac surgery before coming to us and were there to improve their paper qualifications, but their knowledge and interest in congenital heart surgery in children was minimal. We were keen on terminating this rotation system and using the available post to attract candidates from the whole of the UK. We approached the Royal College of Surgeons and the Regional Health Authority to discuss the matter. They called a meeting held at the Institute of Child Health, the academic unit of Great Ormond Street, and we found ourselves heavily outnumbered.

There were three consultants from each adult department versus Marc and myself. Sir Keith Ross and Terence English, later Sir Terence, the college president, participated, and both were our friends and supporters. We stated our case, and then the discussion went round the table. The consultants all repeated that once Great Ormond Street terminated the rotation we would be 'dead' in terms of attracting good candidates, as nobody would want to work in our department. My reply was that we would continue to get excellent overseas candidates. As far as the UK was concerned, we would be able to advertise nationally and select the best candidates from the entire country, rather than from the three London hospitals participating in the rotation. We could thus contribute to training in a broader way.

They wouldn't listen. At one point Marc was ready to give up, as we were two against twelve. He whispered, 'Let's forget it.' But I was adamant. Then Keith and Terence chipped in, suggesting that perhaps we should give the new system a try for a couple of years and see how it went. With their support we won the day.

A further problem we faced was the rationalization of paediatric cardiac services throughout the country. There were forty-one departments of cardiothoracic surgery in the UK, each of them dealing with at least a few children. When I looked at the results, there were huge differences between the departments operating on just a few children and those doing hundreds. For example, the mortality for the closure of ventricular septal defect, a relatively simple operation, was under 10 per cent in four large units treating 60 per cent of all UK children with this defect. By contrast, the mortality in the rest of the small units was 40 per cent.

The paediatric cardiologists and paediatric cardiac surgeons got together to discuss the issue. We knew that we had no chance persuading adult cardiac surgeons that they could not operate on a fourteen-year-old child with an atrial septal defect, so we decided to concentrate on infants – that is, children under the age of one year. We made a proposal to the Department of Health suggesting that just six units in England and Wales operate on infants with congenital heart disease, because Scotland had its own system with a separate Ministry of Health.

After a considerable length of discussion, during which local political factors were considered, a decision was made. Nine supraregional units would receive support, including direct funding from the Department of Health. That was three more units than we had suggested, but it was certainly a major step forward. When I was later preparing my presidential address for the European Association for Cardiothoracic Surgery I was able to demonstrate the results of this rationalization to reduce the number of departments operating on infants with congenital heart defects. The mortality rate in the supraregional centres dropped dramatically, although there remained considerable differences between departments operating on more than 250 children and those operating on fewer than 100.

During the first five to ten years after I left Czechoslovakia for good I had a recurring dream that I was back in Prague. Each time I would ask myself why on earth I had gone back as I would never be able to return to London, and I would wake up sweating and anxious. Another nightmare related to my appointment at Great Ormond Street. When would they discover that 'little Jarda' from Czechoslovakia had landed this wonderful job despite the fact that his training was not up to scratch? Slowly but surely the nightmares stopped, to my relief.

15
LECTURES AND PUBLICATIONS, 1975

I was always enthusiastic about lecturing and writing papers based on my experiences in surgery. During my early years in Czechoslovakia, when I started in Rychnov, I published papers in the Czech surgical journal *Rozhledy v chirurgii*. The first was on the surgical treatment of tennis elbow – although there were precious few tennis players in this mountainous region. The Communist regime forced many white-collar office workers into factory jobs, and the repetitive movements at the assembly line frequently provoked epicondylitis or tennis elbow. I also published a paper on cholecystectomy for acute cholecystitis with early post-operative mobilization of patients. I think that my then boss was the first surgeon to practise this approach in Czechoslovakia.

Later I published and presented papers at meetings in Prague and Bratislava. Cardiac skiing meetings started in Cervinia in Italy and later moved to Courchevel and finally to Val d'Isère. They were thoroughly enjoyable events attended by around thirty to forty participants. One day was dedicated to adult cardiac surgery, a second to congenital problems and the third day was a mixed bag including research and transplantation. We all knew each other well, so there was no standing on ceremony or one-upmanship, and the meetings were well structured. Everybody presented candid results, so our sessions were highly informative and useful. We would generally ski until about 4 p.m., then the meeting proceeded from 5 p.m. until 8.30 p.m., followed by dinner. I remember one year when we ski'ed from Courchevel to Val Thorens two of our American registrars had great difficulty negotiating the slopes of Cime de Caron, a black run. My colleague Gerald Graham, aged sixty-five, was going slowly but surely. He had taught himself to ski at the age of fifty, so he was doing well. The Americans usually did not ski much during their training, as they worked such long and gruelling hours that there was never much time for anything other than work.

STARK CHOICES: FROM PRAGUE TO LONDON AND BEYOND

Another good ski meeting was a combined cardiology and cardiac surgery postgraduate course in Snowmass, Colorado, organized by Bruce Paton, a surgeon from Denver, and John Vogel, a cardiologist from Santa Barbara. John was an enterprising person. One time in London he visited our home with his girlfriend and described how some years before he had climbed up to a mountain hut in the Rockies where he catheterized himself to measure his pulmonary artery pressure, as he had been trying to determine the influence of altitude on PA pressure. I was invited to lecture three times in Snowmass. The programme would start at 8 a.m. and continue until 11.30. Then there was an 'extended lunch break for skiing' until 4.30 in the afternoon. A work session would be followed by dinner and finally a moonlight session after that. Snowmass involved good friends, good skiing and, on the whole, very high-quality presentations.

The first time I attended one of these meetings Bruce Paton collected me from the airport and took me to his family home, where I spent a day with him and his wife. He examined my clothing before driving us to the Rockies to ensure that I had a good anorak. Mine was a very warm one made of goose feathers, but on seeing it he suggested that I borrow one of his instead which he felt would provide better insulation. I was very grateful because when we arrived it was exceedingly cold. The next day I was taken to the top of the mountain where it was around −35 degrees centigrade with the wind-chill factor.

Our group was mainly from Denver, so the others had been skiing for about seven weeks already, while it was the first time that season for me. I told them that I needed to tie my laces and that they should go ahead of me. Once they had disappeared I attempted a few turns on the snow. It felt OK, so I ski'ed down, passing them on the way. At the bottom they were surprised by the speed of my descent and asked me where I skied in London. I told them Hampstead Heath but did not reveal that I had been skiing since the age of two and a half.

In 1975 a very good meeting was organized in Detroit to celebrate twenty-five years of open-heart surgery. It was sponsored by the Henry Ford Foundation. I was invited together with another four or five surgeons from the UK. We were sent first-class tickets, and those of us who wanted to bring their spouses changed their tickets to two economy ones – apart from Lord Brock. He arrived first class, while his wife flew economy. The meeting started with a session on the history of cardiac surgery by Dr Bigelow, Lord Brock and others. I was sitting next to John Kirklin, who whispered to me that the discussion seemed to emanate from a dinosaurs' graveyard.

One of the highlights was Jane Somerville's presentation on pulmonary atresia. The whole meeting was being televised, so there were a lot of bright lights concentrated on the podium and on the speakers. Jane was showing her slides, which were a little fuzzy. She asked for the lights to be dimmed, but nothing happened, so she repeated her request – to no avail. Finally she said in a loud voice, 'Would you please switch the lights off. I prefer it in the dark.' For the rest of the meeting people spoke of nothing but Jane liking it in the dark. This was despite Adib Jatene from Rio de Janeiro presenting his first successful arterial switch operation for transposition of the great arteries, a milestone in paediatric cardiac surgery. Not even this lecture could upstage Jane's remark.

I visited the Detroit Museum of Fine Art with Russian surgeon George Falkovski. We enjoyed a couple of hours in the museum, walking there and back. When we told our American friends they were horrified. We had apparently walked through the most dangerous neighbourhood in Detroit.

I also lectured that year in Toronto, Bergamo, Tegernsee and Washington, DC. The Helen Taussig Symposium on Pediatric Cardiology in Baltimore in 1975 was particularly interesting, commemorating, as it did, her eightieth birthday. I learned some good stories about Dr Taussig. When she realized that blue children with Fallot's tetralogy did better if they had a patent ductus arteriosus she travelled to Boston to see Dr Gross, the first surgeon to close the ductus. She asked him if he would be prepared to create a ductus, rather than ligate one. Dr Gross was indignant. 'Madame, I close PDAs, not create them.' So then she asked her surgeon at Johns Hopkins University, Dr Blalock, who did the first shunt, which was for ever after known as the Blalock–Taussig shunt.

Vivien Leigh was a technician in the animal laboratory at Johns Hopkins. During this meeting he was awarded an honorary doctorate by the university. Apparently one day he came to Dr Blalock and asked him if he wanted to create an atrial septal defect without bypass. Dr Blalock thought that it was impossible, but Vivien showed him how to do it in the dog laboratory. So the Blalock–Hanlon atrial septostomy was born. As for the Blalock–Taussig shunt, Vivien is also credited with having done the first shunt in a laboratory. Dr Taussig used to organize a lunch every year for her residents and interns. Before they could eat they had to work for about forty minutes in her garden. It is related that her chief resident was busy with a patient, so he arrived late. Everybody was eating, but Dr Taussig gave him a shovel to do his half-hour stint in the garden before allowing him his meal.

In 1976 I chaired a session at the European Congress of Cardiology in Amsterdam. The welcome reception was held in the impressive Van Gogh Museum and was most enjoyable. The same year I went as an honorary speaker to a meeting of the Scandinavian Society for Cardiothoracic Surgery in Trondheim. I started my lecture by showing a picture of the Charles Bridge in Prague, because there had been a famous battle there between the Czechs and the Swedes during the Thirty Years War. I commented that I was glad that the hostilities were forgotten since they had invited me to attend. At this point the projector jammed, and it took thirty minutes to obtain a replacement. I started my lecture again by saying that I should be more cautious, as possibly ancient hostile forces were still at work.

A new medical school had been opened in Kuwait. My friend Dr Mohsen Alabdulrazzak Yousef, then dean of the Medical School who was also head of the Department of Cardiology, invited us to the opening ceremony. I was sent two first-class tickets, which Olga and I changed for three economy-class tickets in order to take Jaroslav. First we visited Iran. On the flight from London the pilot made an announcement. He said, 'Ladies and gentleman, we will be landing at Tehran International Airport in one hour thirty minutes exactly – maybe!' I suppose this was his idea of a translation of *inshallah*.

In Tehran we visited a good friend, a former Great Ormond Street resident, Hormoz Azar. He had left Iran to study in the USA for eight years and had then spent a year with us at Great Ormond Street; after that he returned to Tehran. We had a dinner in his house, but even at home he was reluctant to talk freely. The secret service under the Shah was everywhere, and there were many instances of people's conversations being bugged. I asked, 'Hormoz, tell me: is it really?' He comprehended immediately what I was driving at and said yes. I felt it was terrible but no different from living under Communism in Czechoslovakia.

I duly lectured at the university, and Olga, Jaroslav and I visited Tehran with its bazaar and planned to fly to Isfahan, one of the most interesting cities in Iran with great mosques and another famous bazaar. Arriving at the

LECTURES AND PUBLICATIONS, 1975

airport, we were informed that our flight had been cancelled but that they hoped to get us on the next one in around four hours' time. We waited in the airport lounge, talking to a group of expatriates who had been in Iran for several years. They assured us that once we had the boarding passes we would get on board. I was still suspicious, because it reminded me of many similar chaotic situations back in Czechoslovakia. I went to the guard at the gate and asked him if he could let me know just before boarding commenced, and I handed him twenty dollars. We got on the plane, while the expatriates did not. I was not surprised that my bribe had worked, as similar ones had been effective in many similar situations back home.

Isfahan was amazing. We stayed in a former caravanserai where the caravans used to stop overnight on their travels. There were Persian carpets on the floors, on the walls, just about everywhere. Everything was very beautiful, and visiting the bazaar was a great experience. We loved the Persian carpets – Isfahan, Tabriz and others. Surprisingly, we were advised not to buy carpets there because we could get them cheaper in a warehouse at the London docks. We did just that after our return home. We bought two beautiful Isfahans and a Tabriz, which I have to this day. After Isfahan we planned one more stop in Shiraz, the city of the flower gardens. We looked around there, and the following day a young cardiac surgeon took us to visit the ruins of the ancient city of Persepolis, another incredible experience. Then we travelled on to Kuwait, where we stayed in the Sheraton Hotel in a spacious suite. On arrival I was asked to do a clinic the next morning to see some of the children on whom I had operated in London as well as some new patients. They took me back to the hotel at about 2.30 p.m.

The opening ceremony of the new medical school was at 7.30 that evening. A taxi was scheduled to pick us up, but it never arrived. I tried calling the hospital, but there were no English-speaking telephonists on hand, as they had left to attend the ceremony. I tried everything but had no luck. Later that evening Jaroslav, who was watching television, said, 'Daddy, look, I think this is where you should be.' It was a live broadcast from the opening ceremony.

A few hours later I met Mohsen in the lobby and explained what had happened. He told me not to worry. 'Just the bloody Arabs,' he said – and he was a blue-blooded Arab himself. He suggested going to the top floor where there was a fine restaurant. A teapot was in the centre of each table. I wasn't impressed and told the waiter that we didn't want tea with our meal. He smiled. 'No, sir. The teapots contain whisky.'

While we were eating our deserts I noticed Jaroslav's eyes growing bigger and bigger. He pointed to a table not far from ours where an Arab couple were treating some friends to a four-course dinner. They had no sooner finished than they started all over again – the waiter arrived with a huge platter of king prawns. Their friends were reciprocating! This seemed to explain why so many of the Arabs we saw in Kuwait were obese.

The next day Mohsen hosted a dinner in his house for the conference speakers. He seemed somewhat nervous. When I asked why he told me that we were having baked oysters as a starter and that they were best accompanied by whisky but that he wasn't sure if Dr Al-Fagih, a surgeon from Saudi Arabia, was coming. He was a strict Muslim, and, if he attended, there would be no chance of alcohol with our meal. Mohsen reassured me that Al-Fagih was unlikely to arrive so late, but at this point the surgeon walked into the room – so that was the end of our chance of a snifter.

The same year I presented a paper on the surgical treatment of Truncus arteriosus in infancy and another one on the palliative Mustard operation at the meeting of the American College of Cardiology in Las Vegas. I also went to an international symposium on complex congenital heart disease in Milan and chaired a session during the Second European Symposium on Paediatric Cardiology in London.

In 1977 I was invited to the congress of the Brazilian Society of Cardiology in Porto Alegre. I flew to Rio de Janeiro where Paulo, our former resident from Rio, met me. I spent an enjoyable day with him and his boss Milton Meyer. Olga was due to arrive the next day, because she had to make sure that Jaroslav got off to his summer school in Nice. I thought that my hosts would collect her at the airport the next day, as she was due to land at 4 a.m. But they insisted that I come along as well and brought a large bouquet of flowers to greet her. We were put up in a lovely hotel on the border between the Copacabana and the Ipanema Beaches. There was a pool on the top floor with a beautiful view over the sea, while in the other direction, less than two kilometres away, we could see shanty towns built of cardboard and tin. In the evening Paulo and Milton took us to a churrascaria, a wonderful place where they served three kinds of meat on the spit: beef, lamb and bulls' testicles. The waiters kept replenishing our plates. It was a feast. The next day we went to another restaurant where I ordered the smallest possible steak, but it still overlapped my plate by 10 centimetres on each side. My Brazilian friends were not fazed by the portion sizes; they each asked for a doggy bag and took away what would have been enough for lunch for the whole family the following day.

I gave a talk on infant cardiac surgery in the Centro de Estudos de Chirurgia Cardiovascular Infantil, Instituto Estadual do Cardiologia, in Rio de Janeiro. Olga and I went up Corcovado, the mountain from which the great statue of Christ towers over the city, and we also took the funicular up Sugarloaf Mountain, from where we had breathtaking views over the city.

The next day we flew to Porto Alegre, a large city at the southern tip of Brazil. On the way we flew over the famous Iguazu Falls. The pilot tilted the plane for his passenger to see them, then he made another pass and tilted the plane on the other wing.

Porto Alegre is an industrial city with a very large population of Germans. The day after our arrival we were invited to the house of the chief of cardiac surgery, a Dr Ivo Nesrala. I asked him if he had any Czech ancestors. He said no but added that, oddly enough, he had been asked the question many times. The poor man had no idea that the Czech translation of his name was 'no shit'.

During the reception I talked to Dr Zerbini, a famous Brazilian cardiac surgeon, and to Adib Jatene, who did the first arterial switch. Adib was a brilliant surgeon, but he became convinced that he could serve his country better as a politician. So he became Minister of Health. I greatly admired his conviction. After the meeting, at which I presented three papers, we were invited to a farm 100 kilometres from Porto Alegre owned by an orthopaedic surgeon friend of Dr Nesrala. When we arrived, we discovered that a great deal of entertainment had been organized – horse-riding, tennis and swimming – but the main activity was drinking Caipirinha. It tastes innocent enough and is a mixture of cachaça, made from sugarcane, lime and sugar; it's the sugar that makes it lethal. The cachaça there was probably 80 per cent proof, so after two Caipirinhas one was likely to find oneself under the table. The orthopaedic surgeon told us that it was a very small farm but that he owned a bigger one in Mato Grosso. When I asked him how big that one was he said it was about the size of Portugal.

From Porto Alegre we flew to Brasilia, Brazil's capital. It was an interesting flight as the plane flew low to the ground. You could see the endless jungle below. The country is so huge that it took us six hours to get from the southern tip to Brasilia, situated in the north. The city was developed by Lúcio Costa, the principal city planner, and Oscar Niemeyer, the principal architect. It is a formally planned city with schools, churches and ministries divided into different quarters, instead of being developed organically over centuries. This feels rather artificial, even though some of the buildings are phenomenal examples of modern architecture. The locals do not like the new city very much, so most of the bureaucrats and officials fly home to Rio or São Paulo for the weekend, and Brasilia becomes a ghost town. Our visit was an interesting experience, but I am not sure I would like to live there either.

From there we flew to Manaus, where we stayed overnight. The airline's hotel was in the middle of a jungle at the confluence of the Rio Negre and the Amazon river. These two rivers merge into one mammoth one, the Amazon, so broad that you cannot see its opposite bank. It was a lovely place with fabulous tropical birds singing outside our windows. We had remarkably good fish for dinner and went for a walk in the jungle.

Manaus is famous for its opera house, which was built for Maria Callas. We went into the town and witnessed a disturbing incident. Close to the market we saw a young man running along the narrow gap between the stalls. A minute later a lorry with about fifteen soldiers appeared. The soldiers jumped out, chased him, caught him and threw him into the lorry where they kicked him viciously. We learned later about police brutality and heard stories about people disappearing without a trace.

From Manaus we flew to Venezuela to visit Petr (Pedro) Pick, my old friend from primary school in Prague and scouting days. Petr had emigrated from Prague to Venezuela with his parents through a Jewish organization in 1948, just after the Communist takeover. They started with a small business making paints, and Petr weighed the bags. Later, when they had more money, they sent him to study in the USA. He chose Cornell University, because it had a very good tennis team and he was a keen player. Over the next few years he ascended the ranks of his parents' company and was made chief executive. It became one of the largest petrochemical companies in South America, so he was my only millionaire friend. None of this ever changed Petr. Even after so many years it was as if we had seen one other just the day before. Later on, when he and his wife Barbara visited London they usually stayed at the Connaught Hotel, one of the most exclusive and most expensive in town, and we were invited to join them for lovely dinners there. But when we reciprocated Petr was happy to come to a small bistro in Hampstead or a Chinese restaurant in Soho. He was very happy and relaxed wherever we took him.

Petr and Barbara had a lovely house in Caracas with a swimming-pool. When I went to give a lecture at the hospital Olga stayed behind with Barbara who was drinking a Coke by the pool. Olga, who was thirsty, asked for a sip and discovered it was not Coca-Cola but a Cuba libre with far more rum than Coke. We felt Petr and Barbara were drinking too much. Indeed on other occasions, during their visits to our home in London, I would open a bottle of Scotch, of which Olga and I would have a small glass; by the end of the evening there was barely a drop left. On the second or third day of our visit to Caracas Petr complained that his son Tommy, then aged about eighteen, had come home very drunk. Olga and I remarked that we were not surprised because when Tommy saw his parents drinking heavily he would think it was normal to drink to excess. Petr seemed taken aback. He asked if we thought he and Barbara drank too much, and when I replied in the affirmative he said that he would not touch hard liquor from then on but stick to wine only. Olga had a bet with him as to whether he could keep his word, and to our amazement he did. He switched to wine and never touched spirits again.

Some years later I had a call from Petr at Machu Picchu. At the top of the mountain he had developed chest pain. The next day he consulted a cardiologist who told him that there were changes to his electrocardiogram. Petr asked me what he should do. I said that with his undoubted willpower I could not understand why he was still smoking. He asked if it really mattered. When I confirmed that it was a significant factor in heart disease he said that he would never smoke another cigarette again. Once again he kept his word.

His subsequent career was amazing. He organized seminars for top politicians, diplomats and military people. These were usually held for three or four days in a remote place, and the conclusions from the discussions were subsequently sent to the government, ministry or institution that would find them helpful. Later Petr took a three-month course at Boston Business School, which was attended by diplomats, top industrialists and military personnel. It was expensive, but he paid for himself, as he did not want to be in his company's debt. There were a few options he could take after the course. He could become adviser behind the scenes to the Venezuelan president, which might have had unpleasant repercussions for his family, so he decided to leave his job in Caracas and accept a position with Arthur D. Little, a famous consultancy firm. He joined around 1986 on a salary of US $250,000 – which was like pocket-money compared with his income as a chief executive. Within a short time he was running Arthur Little's branches in Boston, Caracas and Prague and became the company's vice-president. Eventually he decided to move to Prague with Barbara. He said that it was better to be 'a big fish in a small pond than a small fish in a big pond'. They lived in a villa near my sister's flat but eventually rented a lovely apartment on the embankment between Charles Bridge and the National Theatre overlooking the castle. He organized several seminars similar to those held in Venezuela called 'Sdružení Lípa'. He invited me to one meeting in Český Krumlov, where our friend Vojta Volavka from the USA introduced a discussion on the abuse of hard drugs. It was a very interesting lecture. Vojta was explaining his experience with heroin, which they were using in diminishing doses to help addicts kick their habit. Vojta had the keys to the safe where the heroin was kept, and one day he tried it himself. He was horrified. After a single dose he had the terrible urge to use it again, so he gave the keys to his colleague, saying that under no circumstances was he to have access to the contents of the safe. I found that fascinating. Sadly Petr was to die prematurely in 2004 of a cerebral lymphoma.

In September 1977 I attended a paediatric cardiology meeting in Boston Children's Hospital and, soon after, a European Cardiac Surgeons' Club meeting in Toledo. We stayed in the parador on the other side of the Tagus river with wonderful views. El Greco must have painted his picture of Toledo from that spot. There is a wonderful collection of El Greco pictures in the cathedral, and the old town itself is a gem. I also lectured around that time in Milan, Sheffield and Munich.

Later Olga and I were invited to the World Congress of Cardiology in Tokyo. Our travel agent arranged first-class tickets at a reasonable price, but we had to fly via Paris. While waiting to board at Charles de Gaulle Airport, I saw on the monitor that the flight to Tokyo was scheduled to go via Moscow and was appalled. I went to the counter and explained that when booking the flight I had specified that we could not fly that route. I was still sentenced to a year in a labour camp in Czechoslovakia, and I had heard of instances where people in my circumstances from the Eastern Bloc countries had been arrested when changing planes in the Soviet Union or in other Iron Curtain countries. The woman at the counter tried to reassure me that going via Moscow was the quickest route, but when I insisted that I would not take it she altered the flight to one the next day. It was difficult to find overnight accommodation at short notice, but we discovered a cheap hotel near the Place Bastille. We suspected it was 'an hourly hotel', and we did not get much sleep what with all the furtive goings-on in adjacent rooms.

In Tokyo we had to walk from the international to the national terminal, as we were flying on to Kyoto. A Tokyo cardiac resident met us at the international airport's arrivals hall. He bowed, took my suitcase from me, marched ahead and never looked back. I wanted to take Olga's suitcase, but she said no, as she wanted to see his reaction to her struggling with heavy baggage, but the man was unconcerned. That was the way things were in Japan. It was curious, because he had spent two years in Germany and should have been familiar with European ways. In Kyoto we stayed in a very comfortable *ryokan*, a typical Japanese bed-and-breakfast. After the tour of the city we visited Nara, the ancient capital of Japan before Kyoto and Tokyo, where Dr Shigehito Miki was in charge of cardiac surgery. He had spent about eight years with Donald Ross in London and visited us a few times at Great Ormond Street. He invited me to give a talk in Nara. We had an excellent lunch in the centre of a large park with many deer. It was in a traditional restaurant, where they cook everything in front of you on a hotplate built into the centre of the table.

My lecture in the hospital was translated by an interpreter sentence by sentence, so it took ages. We were very late for dinner, which was also to be a traditional Japanese affair. Olga meanwhile had been taken out for the afternoon by two wives of local surgeons. When she asked them what a traditional Japanese dinner involved they said they did not know; they had never been invited to one. Yet both were graduates of Kyoto University, the Japanese equivalent of Oxbridge. The three women arrived at the restaurant but were refused admission, as it was men only. The two Japanese resolved the situation by promoting Olga to 'honorary man', as the wife of an important English professor. It worked. They got in and were drinking tea

103

when we finally arrived two hours later. Olga, with typical sardonic humour, said, 'We are not sure if we want you men here. You're very late.' This went down like a lead balloon.

When we sat down to dinner, the establishment's head geisha was in charge of proceedings. She was an elderly woman, about sixty and versatile in music, poetry and the art of social conversation. I was assigned a trainee geisha, about sixteen years old, who sat between Olga and me. She was somewhat shy for the first ten minutes, but after that she embarked on entertaining me. She poured sake into my cup, attempted to make conversation with about ten words of English and flirted with me. My wife and I knew that geishas were entertainers not prostitutes, but it was remarkable to observe her ignoring Olga completely. Olga meanwhile spent the evening talking to one of the surgeon's wives and had fun surreptitiously observing the young girl.

In Tokyo the daughter of the President of the Congress was our guide. She was a very pleasant young woman of about twenty-four who spoke excellent English and who worked for a foreign company. She told us the old traditions were still strong in Japan and that her parents were hoping to marry her off with the assistance of a match-maker, which she very much resented. She got in touch with us a few years later, and we discovered that she was still not married.

We visited Osaka where I gave a guest lecture at the Asia Heart Centre and spent a night in the head surgeon's house. The rooms were bare, and we slept on tatamis on the floor. As there were no wardrobes or chests we wondered where people kept their clothes and other possessions. The house was small, and there seemed to be no storage space anywhere. It was another example of the cultural difference between the East and the West in those days.

16
TRAVELS, 1979–1982, AND A VISIT TO CHINA

In 1979 I participated in another Snowmass 'skiing conference', after which I went as a visiting professor to the Mayo Clinic. Then I flew via Milwaukee to Toronto. I had been having problems with my knee, and Bill Marshall, a microbiologist from Great Ormond Street who was a sports doctor for several London soccer clubs, had examined me. He concluded that it was a 'typically atypical meniscus injury'! He recommended that his good friend in Canada, an orthopaedic physician, do an arthroscopy on me. When I corresponded with his friend he told me that if he found something wrong with the meniscus he would refer me to Dr Jackson, an orthopaedic surgeon in Toronto who was the only surgeon doing meniscetomies arthroscopically. He suggested that I go straight to Dr Jackson, so I arranged to consult him after my visit to the Mayo Clinic.

When I arrived in Milwaukee the airport was closing because of a snowstorm. My flight was badly delayed, so I arrived in Toronto very late and reached the hospital at around midnight. I thought that no way would I have my operation the next morning. But at about 12.30 that night Dr Jackson came to see me. He apologized for the delay, saying that because of the heavy snow it had been difficult for him to get to the hospital earlier. He examined me and confirmed that he would do an arthroscopy and, if need be, take the meniscus out at 8.30 that morning. When I was coming round from the anaesthesia the next day he turned up. He asked if I had any problems walking. I explained that I had not yet woken up so I had not tried to walk. He told me, 'You'd better get on your bike. If you want to fly to London tomorrow, you better get in some practice walking.' I did – and I flew to London the next day!

In March, just six weeks after my knee operation, I decided to participate in the giant slalom competition at our skiing meeting in Cervinia. I had read that basketball players were back on the pitch a week after arthroscopic meniscetomies, so I thought that I could ski six weeks later. Of course the basketball players were very fit 25-year-olds – and I was forty-five. Nevertheless I ski'ed well, and through the last three gates I was skating to gain additional speed. Unfortunately I edged the skis and fell. As a result I came third – a major disappointment for someone as competitive as me.

I also attended the Society of Thoracic Surgeons meeting in Phoenix and a symposium on problems in paediatric cardiology in Padua, where I received a special commemorative medal from the university. I also visited Seville, Madrid, Amsterdam, Hanover and Bangkok. In the summer I participated at the Great Ormond Street annual two-week course on paediatric cardiology and cardiac surgery in Cambridge, with a surgeon, a cardiologist and a pathologist in residence all the time. About forty doctors, mainly from Europe but some from further overseas, participated. Lecturers and participants went out to local pubs each night. One of the lecturers was Jim Wilkinson, a cardiologist from Liverpool who was a very entertaining man who could mimic any accent. We had some hilarious evenings. He later emigrated to Australia and became the head of a paediatric cardiology unit at the Royal Melbourne Children's Hospital, and some years later he was my host there.

In 1979 I was invited to China to strengthen the ties between British and Chinese cardiac surgeons. This was an initiative of Dr Zhu, who had spent six months at Great Ormond Street and a further six months in Leeds with Marian Ionescu. Subsequently he climbed the ladder of the Chinese Academy of Medical Sciences so was in a position to extend the invitation to me and another surgeon. It was somewhat ironic that the two representing Britain were Jaroslav Stark from Czechoslovakia and Marian Ionescu from Romania, but this time there were many foreign medics performing at the top level in Britain.

I wrote to Beijing and asked what topics they would like me to prepare for my lectures and suggested a dozen. Back came the answer: 'All twelve please.' We flew to Hong Kong. Marian had developed the Ionescu–Shiley valve, so the Shiley company invited us to a dinner in the Hong Kong Sheraton. The food was delicious, and after the starter they served a sorbet to cleanse the palate. Marian's wife Christina was a cardiologist in Leeds but rarely attended functions with her husband. She was indignant, telling the waiter that she had not ordered ice cream, especially not so early during the meal.

From Hong Kong we took a train to Canton (Guangzhou) from where we were supposed to fly to Peking (Beijing) that day, but the plans had changed. We were taken to a hotel and told that we would now fly the following morning. We had time to explore the city that afternoon. We went to see a flower show, which was spectacular. Some plants had as many as 2,000 flowers, and some of the stems were trained into remarkable shapes. The horticulturists were especially proud of their bonsai trees. We dined in the evening in a very good restaurant with typical Cantonese food. The ground floor was for people who were paying, as opposed to the first floor which was for guests for whom the dinner had been arranged and paid for by their hosts. This was a Communist idea of equality! Next day we took a taxi to the airport. This was scary, because people drove very fast and far too close to the hundreds of cyclists. The driver hooted continuously but managed not to knock anyone down.

Our visit to China took place not long after the Cultural Revolution. At Beijing Airport we were met by a welcoming committee: Dr Zhu and the head of the medical section of the Academy, several interpreters and a few others. They gave us a print-out of our programme for the next week and suggested that we went to the hotel to discuss and 'criticize the programme'. We headed for the Friendship Hotel, a vast building constructed in the 1950s for visiting Soviet experts assisting China. The first item on the programme was a visit to the Forbidden City, followed the next day by preparations for operations to be conducted by me and the third day three open-heart procedures 'by Mr Stark'. This took me by surprise, as in our correspondence there had been no mention of my doing any surgery. However, I did not feel like criticizing anything. The atmosphere was tense and reminded me of the worst years of the Communist regime in Czechoslovakia.

We enjoyed our walk through the Forbidden City and Tiananmen Square. Olga sprang ahead excitedly. 'Is that Mao's mausoleum over there?' she enquired. As our interpreter-cum-minder accompanied her to the mausoleum it gave me five minutes with the doctors on my own. Olga and I developed this tactic and similar ones to talk to Chinese colleagues privately, because we feared that everything we discussed was being overheard and noted. Even in our hotel room we did not feel safe to talk freely, as we felt sure there were hidden listening devices. Even when we were on our own we did not talk about anything potentially incriminating. When we met Dr Zhu the next day I told him that I brought him as a gift a copy of my book and that I would bring it to the hospital. 'Please don't. It will be confiscated for the hospital library. I will come to your hotel to collect it later,' he said.

The following day we had a seminar to discuss the three patients on whom I was to operate. The first one was a two-year-old child with ventricular septal defect, a simple hole in the heart. He had had cardiac catheterization but no angiogram. This had not been carried out, as there was not enough money to perform the procedure on every patient. From the history and from the catheterization data it was fairly clear to me that the ventricular septal defect was closing and that the child did not need an operation now or possibly ever. After I conveyed my professional opinion there was a long silence. Despite my advice the medics remained adamant. 'You will operate tomorrow morning.' I presumed this was the child of a party official and that the parents had been promised surgery. I kept quiet, thinking that perhaps it was preferable for me to operate on the child rather than the local surgeons. They asked me what I required for the procedure. They seemed somewhat embarrassed, because when I asked about anaesthesia and perfusion they seemed to have very little clue. However I went to theatre and with the help of a scrub nurse selected a few instruments.

I operated the next day while Olga went to the children's hospital to lecture on congenital rubella. The technicians could not find the cannulae I had selected the previous day, and the cardioplegia needle was very blunt, but that was all they had. They did not have a suitable retractor for the tricuspid valve, but we improvised. As I anticipated, we found a small ventricular septal defect which was easily closed with a direct suture. The scrub nurses were very good and soon learned to read my gestures when I required forceps, scissors or other surgical implements. So the operation went smoothly, and the child did well.

The second operation was on a ten-year-old boy with Fallot's tetralogy. He was not blue but black! His haemoglobin was 26 grams per cent (the normal range being 12–14 grams per cent). The operation was fairly straightforward, but when we came off bypass the child's blood pressure was low. I asked for an adrenaline drip, which was at that time our catecholamine of choice to raise blood pressure. After a while I looked up and could not see the drip. So I repeated my request – this time more urgently. They said that the drip was up. I could see only a large cylinder containing perhaps three litres of blood, which was dripping fast. I was told that the adrenaline was in the blood. In despair I asked how much adrenaline in micrograms per kilogram of body weight the child was receiving. The anaesthetist asked the nurses, 'What's the weight of the child?'

Despite such hurdles everything went fine. We reused gloves that were washed after being used on a previous patient. These were put into disinfectant and used again and again. For the line from the heart–lung machine to the patient they had a series of short tubes connected together, as there was not enough money to purchase a single long tube. Everything clearly required considerable improvisation. At the end of surgery the operating staff would not allow me to close the chest and took me out for tea, while they closed the chest themselves.

There was, in fact, a third patient scheduled for surgery with me that day. When I examined the child, aged about fourteen years, I found he had extremely bad teeth. I explained during the seminar that this problem had to be addressed first; only after the teeth had been dealt with could the boy undergo major heart surgery. So I performed just two operations that day.

I suggested starting my lectures earlier in the day than scheduled because there were three topics to cover. This was not possible, as lunch had already been arranged. I assumed this would be a light meal, but, no, we had five courses and each was extremely good. I discovered that the Chinese are very fond of their food. On finishing our lunch we got to the lecture hall and found that the audience had just left for theirs. We then had to wait another forty-five minutes before starting. The lectures were translated sentence by sentence, which I found extraordinarily tedious as it was hard to maintain one's train of thought. It took ages, and at the end I felt exhausted.

The next item on the agenda was a visit to the Great Wall. Our hosts asked us to be ready by 8 a.m., but I wanted to go to the hospital early in the morning to see the second patient on whom I had operated the previous day. They could not comprehend this. I was the surgeon; the operation was over; so why bother going? But they took me to see the boy anyway. He had bled just 250 millilitres overnight. I was amazed. If I had operated on such a blue patient in London whose pre-operative haemoglobin was 26 grams per cent he would have bled at least 800–1000 millilitres post-operatively. I was not sure what Chinese medicine they used to control the bleeding, but it worked superbly well.

We then drove out to the Great Wall, which was spectacular. It was a sunny day, and we had an excellent view of the man-made structure, which I believe is the only one on earth that can be seen from space. I was told it was constructed by 6.5 million workers. As we walked to the top we met a number of ethnic groups in their national costumes, and our cameras were kept busy. On the way back from the wall we visited the Ming Tombs – also a fascinating experience.

Fu Wai Children's Hospital was next on our list. It has the largest unit for surgery of congenital heart defects in China. On the steps of the hospital we were welcomed by five leading consultants holding a large placard with Chinese characters that read, 'Welcome, Dr and Mrs Stark'. We were taken to a large room where the hospital's director gave a welcome speech and told us about the history of the institution and their plans for the future. They had eight wards, each with forty children, but they also had a department of traditional Chinese medicine. Apparently there were three medical schools in Beijing: one taught Western medicine, one Chinese traditional medicine and the third used Western research techniques to find out why Chinese medicine worked. The intensive care unit had three beds, each with a glass cylinder drip and lid. If they wanted to add medication to the drip they simply took the cover off and poured it in. This struck me as highly unusual, as sterility is crucial and normally everything is sealed in a closed system.

During our visit to the children's hospital we were shown around by an orthopaedic surgeon who interpreted for us. His English was excellent despite the fact that he had never been abroad. Congenital surgery had been started there in August 1978 by a woman surgeon, Dr Ma Ru Po, although lack of equipment was always a major problem. We were somewhat surprised that they were developing congenital heart surgery at the hospital, since this requires so much equipment and is generally very expensive. Their rationale was simple: they said that people seeing blue children were distressed and wanted something done about it; other diseases might be less evident, and therefore there was less pressure to treat them.

It was good that we had time to look around Beijing. The Forbidden City was amazing from the point of view of its architecture and sculpture. We started at the Gate of Divine Pride, then visited the museum. There were exhibits of wonderful jewellery, some with precious stones cut for the coronation of emperors, many others in stunningly carved jade. Turtles, the symbols of longevity, were executed magnificently in bronze. The Palace of Earthly Tranquillity and the Hall of Union were especially memorable. We found the marble decoration there, about 30 metres long, immensely impressive; it had been transported to Beijing from a distance of about 800 kilometres. One of the palaces, according to our interpreter, was known as the Palace of Peaceful Intercourse. Certainly the ceiling there had the most exquisite decorations! Finally, through another outside gate, we reached Tiananmen Square. From the balcony above the square Mao had proclaimed the Republic in 1949.

The President of the Chinese Academy of Medical Sciences invited us to a banquet in Heavenly Peaceful Duck, an excellent Pekinese restaurant. The president was an elderly man who had studied literature in the USA. Toasts of '*Jiangkhang*' accompanied the consumption of a fiery liquor called Maotai, which is strong enough to burn one's throat. Fortunately the formal banquets are usually speedy affairs. We started at 6.30 p.m. and finished at about 8.30, despite the fact that we ate some eighteen different courses. Such a meal is usually concluded with soup, a signal that people can get up and leave.

The next day was reserved for my lectures. It was not easy, as again they were translated sentence by sentence. As before, it was hard to maintain one's train of though and to determine how much the audience had taken in.

The last day, before leaving for Shanghai, Marian and I were keen to provide a banquet for our hosts. We had asked an interpreter the best way to express our thanks, and he said without hesitation, 'A good meal.' As we did not know much about Beijing's restaurants we asked if he would organize it. Being a practical man he enquired as to our food preferences and how much we wanted to spend. We suggested Szechuan, as we had had Peking duck at the opening-ceremony dinner. We asked how much such a banquet was likely to cost, and he reckoned between £20 and £60 per person. It seemed quite a lot of money, so we chose a mid-range price of £40 per head. It turned out that all the private rooms in the Szechuan restaurant were booked, so our next idea was to take a large table in the main restaurant, but this apparently was not acceptable. You cannot invite people to a banquet unless it is held in a private room. We settled on the Peking Duck, one of Beijing's most famous restaurants.

In the afternoon I received a call from the British consul who told me that he had received a message from the Foreign Office to say that we were in Beijing and asked whether he could be of assistance. I explained that we were leaving the following morning but suggested he could join us for the banquet. 'Jolly good. My wife and I would be delighted to come.' I was vaguely optimistic that the Consulate might help us pay for the meal. No way. The couple just wanted to have a good time – and they did. His wife downed one glass of Maotai after another – and told me later that it was more or less pure alcohol so you wouldn't get a hangover. In the event, the food was superb, and as a co-host I served guests sitting to my right and left with extra-long chopsticks. When I successfully managed to serve slippery mushrooms it seemed my technique in this respect was appreciated far more than my lecturing or operating skills. After we had been eating for half an hour or so I asked the person next to me how far we had gone through the menu. He pointed to the first line indicating the hors d'oeuvre!

Next morning we left for Shanghai. Sitting in the lounge at the airport we saw two old Russian Antonov planes, and Olga insisted that she would not fly in one. Fortunately when they called us for boarding around the corner was a bright new Boeing 707. We flew with Chia, our interpreter-cum-minder, who was a very courteous and intelligent young man. He had worked for a few years as a barefoot doctor. They are educated in the basic principles of hygiene, medicine, nursing and first aid and work in villages where there is no doctor. By educating the villagers in proper use of clean water, in diagnosing simple conditions such as appendicitis and sending patients to hospital where necessary, they performed a valuable service. Chia had been very successful as a barefoot doctor and had thus been selected by the Chinese Academy to study English and become its official interpreter.

Marian and Christina did not travel with us to Shanghai because they were returning to London early. After arriving there we were assigned a second interpreter: a young woman who had served in the Red Guard during the Cultural Revolution. She was a fervent if narrow-minded revolutionary in her attitudes, in total contrast to Chia whom we found to be a mild-mannered, considerate and thoughtful individual.

We received the same welcome in Shanghai as in Beijing. A committee met us at the airport, presented us with the programme for the next few days and suggested that we discuss and 'criticize' it. The first thing I noticed was that they had arranged for me to undertake surgery on the third day. They wanted me to do three operations for the correction of Fallot's tetralogy in infants. At that time in London we were doing this operation in two stages: the shunt in infancy and correction after eighteen to twenty-four months.

By now I felt I had some grasp of Chinese politics. It seemed similar to the form of Communism I had experienced in my youth. So when we arrived at the hotel I said that I had a few criticisms of the planned programme. Everyone froze, as they had not expected this – but they were prepared to listen. I told them that we had been in China for ten days and so far we had not seen a commune, which I understood was one of the major achievements of modern China. I said that I was not sure how I would respond if on my return to London I was asked by members of the working class, 'Comrade, tell us about the communes.' I therefore suggested a modification to the programme. The day I was scheduled to operate I proposed to cancel the surgery and visit a commune instead. I was pretty sure that they would be unable to find any valid counter-argument. And I was right. They agreed to take us to a commune.

Our hotel on the Bund, Ching Chang, was very luxurious, as this was where they billeted the government delegations. In the afternoon Dr Pan Shi, the chief cardiac surgeon, took us on a boat trip on the river. The local river and the Yangtze merge at this point and flow into the sea. During this trip we met Dr Chang, who had been at Great Ormond Street three years earlier. It was somewhat embarrassing that I did not immediately recognize him; fortunately he recalled us immediately, as Olga and I had invited him to dinner at our home in London. In any event he was very good-natured about it.

The next day we left for the commune. Dr Pan Shi was in one taxi with Olga and me, while our two interpreters were in the other vehicle. This meant we had a chance to talk. I presumed that the surgeon guessed that our driver did not understand English, but even so he was careful in what he said. At one point he mentioned that during the Cultural Revolution he was the only cardiac surgeon left in Shanghai, which at that time had well over 15 million inhabitants. When Olga and I exchanged glances, he realized that we had jumped to the conclusion that he must have been a Communist apparatchik. He said no, it was not like that. He explained that his wife had been sent to a commune in the far north-east and his daughter to one in the north-west. He then added the curious remark that his son was lucky as he had gone into the army. Again Olga and I exchanged fleeting looks. He continued, 'From the army one eventually comes back', implying that one rarely returned from a commune.

The commune we saw had about 30,000 people living there. They were self-sufficient, producing everything for themselves. This included agricultural products, farm animals and fisheries. They made steel and had large numbers of carpenters. The children were placed in residential nurseries, where they were well cared for but also protected from 'the potentially bad influence of their parents'. They had a hospital where four barefoot doctors worked. There was a small operating theatre, where they undertook minor surgery such as appendicectomies, hernia repairs and tonsillectomies, all conducted mainly under acupuncture anaesthesia. One of the barefoot doctors explained to us about traditional herbs and their uses. I was particularly impressed with Dr Pan Shi, the Shanghai surgeon, for what he had achieved and as an individual, so subsequently I proposed him for membership of the Society of Thoracic Surgeons, one of the most prestigious American associations of cardiothoracic surgeons. To my delight he was accepted.

The next day I had to give a very long lecture scheduled to last for around three hours. I divided the subjects into three sections, with five minutes' break between each. Once again they translated everything sentence by sentence. The topics were well received, and we had a useful discussion. On the last night of our stay in Shanghai we were invited to dinner by the city's minister of health. It was a small party including the minister, Dr Pan Shi, our interpreter Chia, our Red Guard interpreter, Olga and myself. During the dinner the minister was talking about the difficulties she faced looking after the population not only of Shanghai but of the entire region. When I asked the size of the region's population she replied, 'Altogether, around 250 million people.'

Later on during the course of the meal I felt confident enough to venture a controversial question. I enquired as to whether my hosts could explain how it was possible that Chairman Mao had allowed some of the excesses of the Cultural Revolution. There followed a dead silence. It was as if I had placed a small atom bomb on the table. Finally our interpreter Chia answered, without deferring to the minister or to Dr Pan Shi. He said that we must see the situation in its historical content. For example, he said, look at the French Revolution. In history it is considered a progressive event, yet many terrible things happened during and after in the name of revolution. I was most impressed. After that the discussion once more became friendly and animated.

From Shanghai we flew on to Canton (Guangzhou). Chia, our interpreter, told us that sadly he couldn't accompany us there, as he had been recalled to Beijing. It was a pity, because he had been a wonderful interpreter and companion. We said goodbye and thanked him for everything. At Canton Airport we were greeted by Dr Dong, who had met us off the train from Hong Kong at the beginning of our trip. He took us to Canton's museum of antiquities. Sadly there was little to see there, as so much had been destroyed during the Cultural Revolution by the Red Guards. However, the view from the top of the museum was wonderful, and we enjoyed visiting the Orchid Gardens. Soon after our return to London Olga and I went to the British Museum. We were told that there was a far better collection of Chinese vases and porcelain there than anywhere in China.

I asked Dr Dong, while we were in Canton, for assistance with a cough, which seemed to be developing into tracheitis, as I had a couple of lectures scheduled. I was offered traditional Chinese medicine: bile of snake and ground seashells. I was told that it should be effective but that if I did not improve within twenty-four hours I should try ampicillin – which I eventually did. I gave my two lectures the following day, and the day after we flew to Hong Kong, then via Bangkok back to London.

In 1980 the meeting of the European Cardiac Surgeons' Club was held at Lake Como in Italy. The lake provided a beautiful setting and, as usual, it was an excellent meeting. Meanwhile in June that year London hosted the World Congress of Paediatric Cardiology, where I chaired a session and presented a paper on neonatal cardiac surgery. I was also involved in the London Symposium on Cardioplegia and the European Congress of Cardiology in Paris.

In August 1980 I was invited to a Congress of the Southern African Society of Cardiology in Johannesburg. It was my first visit to the country. Before going we had some heated arguments with Jaroslav. At that time he was

115

studying at Cambridge, was very left-wing and strongly opposed to apartheid, so he opposed my trip. Around that time Olga and I wondered if one day he would come home a card-carrying member of the Communist Party; fortunately he did not. For two rather difficult years Olga was very patient, talking to Jaroslav about the downside of totalitarian regimes for hours. Jaroslav joined the British Labour Party at one point, but he eventually became an independent candidate as a student representative on the University Council – and he won.

I myself was naturally very much opposed to apartheid, so I suggested that Jaroslav should come to South Africa with me, because I wanted to see how it was at first hand. That pacified him somewhat, but in the event he was unable to accompany me. Instead, he demonstrated with fellow students and threw stones outside the South African Embassy in London in protest against that country's racist political regime.

My first impression of South Africa was shocking. I already knew a bit about the place from Amrit Darjee, a houseman in our department, when I first came from Prague to London. He was an Indian from South Africa, and he had told me quite a lot about the iniquitous system there, such as medical personnel not being allowed to transfuse blood from a black person to a white patient. After arriving at the airport in Johannesburg I went to the toilet. A black man was standing next to me. He said quietly, 'Sir, do you realize you are in the wrong toilet?' I said I was sorry that I had not realized but as I was desperate I hoped he would not mind me having a pee there. He said that *he* did not mind but was concerned that I might object to *him* being there. I was shocked. Later on I found that the benches in the parks were labelled 'Whites only' and was disturbed by other evidence of segregation and discrimination. I was also upset by the attitude of some of my South African colleagues from Great Ormond Street who attended the meeting with me. Back in London they presented themselves as true liberals, while in Johannesburg they seemed very right-wing and pro-apartheid, which surprised me greatly.

After the meeting I joined Alain Carpentier and his wife Sophie to visit Londolozi Game Reserve. Alain had operated on a relative of the park manager, and we received wonderful hospitality there in return. Our accommodation was in well-furnished bungalows, and we went for two rides into the reserve: one in the morning, the other in the evening. In the two days we spent there we saw the 'big five': lion, leopard, buffalo, elephant and rhinoceros. It was a wonderful experience.

I then flew to Cape Town for two days. I had been keen to visit this city, and during the meeting in Johannesburg I had promised the Cape Town paediatric cardiologists that I would give a talk on transposition surgery. They offered to organize it in the Red Cross Children's Hospital. Before the lecture they told me that Christiaan Barnard, the surgeon who had performed the first heart transplantation, sent his apologies because he had to go to the dentist for emergency treatment. At any rate my lecture went down well, and afterwards the cardiologists suggested that we go to one of Chris Barnard's restaurants for lunch.

It seemed that he owned three Italian restaurants. When we arrived he was not in fact at the dentist's but was sitting at a table doing his accounts. He was highly embarrassed, so lunch was on the house. I must say I was rather disappointed by him in several ways. He used to come to London to visit David Waterston and learn about children's surgery. He was undoubtedly a very good surgeon, but the number of children on whom he had operated was relatively small. David always treated him with great courtesy, but a few years after Barnard has performed his first heart transplant he gave a lecture on the subject at the Institute of Child Health in Great Ormond Street, and neither David nor I received an invitation.

In September 1980 I was invited to a meeting of the Japanese Society of Cardiac Surgeons in Tokyo. All the street names in the city were in Japanese, so I could not venture outside the hotel alone as I knew I would get lost in no time, but after my lecture I was presented with a generous gift by the society – the latest and most expensive model of Nikon camera. I was thrilled, but when going through customs at Heathrow on my return I declared it, as I naïvely believed that being a gift it would not be taxed. This was a mistake: I had to pay 30 per cent of the camera's value on the spot.

In 1981 Olga and I went to Hershey in Pennsylvania where Dr John Waldhausen had invited me to be visiting professor. Indeed he had been indirectly responsible for me getting the Great Ormond Street job. When he accepted the chairmanship in Hershey he left Philadelphia and Iain Aberdeen left Great Ormond Street to replace him. Iain's consultant post at Great Ormond Street thus became vacant, and I was eventually appointed. John was a very kind host, and we had a very good time together both professionally and socially. During the same trip I was a guest lecturer in Philadelphia, and I also presented five papers at the Symposium on Current Controversies and Techniques in Congenital Heart Surgery in Baltimore.

In addition I attended a meeting of the Catalan Society of Cardiothoracic Surgery in Barcelona. I knew a bit of Spanish, but for the beginning of my lecture I learned the introduction in Catalan. My good friend Marcos Murtra wrote it down for me, we rehearsed it together, and this went down very well.

The American Association for Thoracic Surgery meeting of 1981 was held in Washington, DC. The same year I attended the International Symposium on Arterial Switch Operation in Bergamo, as well as a symposium on Biological Glue in Cardiac Surgery in Hanover, and in December I lectured in Providence and in Boston.

The same year I was appointed to the Ospedale Pediatrico Bambino Gesù in Rome as honorary consultant. The other two honorary consultants were Aldo Castaneda from the Boston Children's Hospital and Anton Becker, a professor of pathology from Amsterdam.

I also presented papers in Bordeaux, Padua and Belgrade. At the end of the year I lectured in Stockholm, where I attended a joint meeting of the European, British and Scandinavian societies of cardiovascular surgery and spoke on surgery for corrected transposition. It was a busy period.

For three years I had been invited to Bombay. Eventually in 1982 I agreed to attend a symposium there. In the letter of confirmation I received I was told the Indian Society had a small budget, so they hoped I would be prepared to pay my own air fare. I felt a certain obligation to attend, so I agreed to this, and I was put up in the impressive Taj Mahal Palace Hotel. However, outside in the street were a great number of beggars – mainly one-legged men or young children. It was a sight I found upsetting every time I left the hotel.

The meeting itself was disappointing. When it came to the important congenital symposium, to which several other speakers from around the world had been invited, I was stunned. There were eight speakers and just ten people sitting in the audience. It seemed an incredible waste of resources.

17
ICELANDIC CONNECTION, 1981

For more than fifteen years we operated on all children with congenital heart defects from Iceland. The population there was about 300,000, so there were only about ten children with heart defects born every year. It would not have been economical to have a fully operational congenital heart unit in that country.

In 1981 Arni Kristinsson, a cardiologist from Reykjavik, sent me and my colleague the consultant cardiologist James Taylor an invitation to give some lectures and spend a week in Iceland. Before we left Arni phoned to suggest I include a dark suit in my luggage. I presumed he was anticipating my participation in one or two formal occasions during our trip.

Soon after our arrival I tried to call Arni but realized I did not have his phone number. I looked in the Reykjavik directory but could not find him. Later I discovered that names in Iceland are unusual; people are named as sons or daughters of their fathers. So Arni Kristinsson's children would not be called Kristinsson but Arnisson or Arnidóttir. Eventually I found him in the directory, where he was listed under the name of Arni!

In the evening Olga and I and James, Anne and their four sons had dinner at the hotel. As a starter we had gravadlax, salmon marinaded in a delicious dill sauce. When we finished our very generous portions the waiter came and offered us second helpings. I had never experienced that before in a hotel restaurant.

After our lectures James and I were informed that the next day we would have an audience with Iceland's Madam President, Vigdís Finnbogadóttir. So I donned my suit, and we presented ourselves at the presidential palace at 9 a.m. The residence was slightly smaller in size than our house in London. James arrived with his whole family, so it took a while to find enough extra chairs. The president was very charming, however, and thanked us for the help we had provided over the years to her nation's children and presented us with the Order of the Falcon, the Icelandic equivalent of a knighthood.

After the audience with the president we rented a car and toured around. We took the main road around the island. Most of it was a dirt track, which after the rain revealed its many potholes. The countryside was amazing, as most of it consisted of lava fields. We were told that before the landing on the moon the cosmonauts had trained near Reykjavik because the landscape there was so similar to the moon.

Every village displayed a sign with its name and the number of inhabitants. Usually it consisted of an unpronounceable name and around thirty-five inhabitants – sixty if it was a large settlement. We visited Thingvellir, the site of the first parliament in Europe. We also saw the hot springs that supplied all the hot water and central heating for the city of Reykjavik at the time. Although it was August we did not remove our two layers of sweaters and wellington boots for the entire holiday, but we had a very enjoyable time.

When we returned to London and Olga mentioned the Order of the Falcon to her boss in microbiology, Professor Dudgeon, he was intrigued. He was one of the old guard with a distinguished military career, and when we met he enquired if I had written to the queen about the award. When I expressed bemusement he told me that I couldn't wear the insignia of a foreign honour without Her Majesty's express permission. I replied that I had no intention of parading my Icelandic knighthood, but he said that that was not the point. If I wrote to her I would get a personal letter from the queen. So partially to please him I agreed to do so and asked if he would compose the letter on my behalf, which he did. And, indeed, three weeks later I had a missive from Her Majesty saying that nothing would give her greater pleasure then if I would wear the insignia of a Knight of the Falcon on all official occasions. I still have the letter.

18
THE NEW CARDIAC WING, 1978–1987

The facilities for the cardiac work we undertook at Great Ormond Street Hospital were, to say the least, inadequate. Originally they consisted of a ward called 1A with twenty beds – six in one bay, four in another and ten single-bed cubicles. Next to this was a catheterization laboratory. Later on we transformed two cubicles into a two-bed intensive care unit. When we acquired another ten beds we used them for pre-operative or convalescing patients prior to discharge. Our offices, which were very small, were located in Barry Wing, a prefab building located on the roof of ward IA. There was an office for David Waterston and Iain Aberdeen. Between the two in a tiny space sat Barbara Grey, their secretary. Dick Bonham Carter and his secretary had an office together, and there was another one for the four registrars – three surgical and one medical. In addition there was a research office and a library used for departmental meetings and joint cardiac conferences. We also had storage for angiograms.

We pleaded with the Department of Health for money to build a purpose-built cardiac unit. Negotiations over this took many years, but in the end they agreed. In 1968 we started to plan our new home, which in itself was very hard work. The main people involved were Ted Battersby, a consultant anaesthetist, James Taylor, the consultant cardiologist, Adelaide Tunstill, our head nurse, and myself. Final approval was received in April 1977, with a projected completion date of June 1980, and work commenced in November 1978. The chairman of the building committee was D.I. Williams, a consultant urologist who proved an outstanding chairman. He discussed everything beforehand, and meetings were swift. When he retired Bill Glover, a consultant anaesthetist, took over the job. Bill was pleasant enough, but his skills as chairman were less adroit. Meetings went on and on, and decisions got delayed. We struggled to keep within our budget, which was

£1 million for the entire project. I managed to get hold of plans for the cardiac units in Boston, the Mayo Clinic and Birmingham, Alabama, and we were able to adapt some of their ideas in a limited way because of NHS financial constraints.

I recall some very tense sessions with the building committee and later on with the commissioning committee. Revised plans were produced on a new scale. They were delivered on a Friday, with all comments to be presented by the following Monday. On perusing them I realized that the architects had omitted a section of offices on the ground floor. I presented my concerns at the Monday meeting, and the plans were duly amended – although rumours went around the hospital that Mr Stark had tried to pull a fast one by adding several extra surgical offices for the unit.

The next problem was deciding on the size of the intensive therapy unit (ITU). Having visited some top units around the world I wanted plenty of space. The addition of a ventilator, extracorporeal membrane oxygenation or a dialysis machine required considerable space. When the ITU was first built the empty space looked enormous, but once it was occupied by beds and equipment one realized that it was the right size.

While cement was being poured into the pilings an elderly clerk of works questioned the adequacy of the amount being used. He felt that it was not sufficient, and on raising his concerns the plans were duly checked. As far as the engineers were concerned, there was no problem – and the clerk of works' concerns were dismissed as those of an old fool.

But the plans had been drawn up wrong. Moreover, astoundingly, a mathematical error of a decimal point had been made when calculating the foundation depth. During the night of 29–30 July 1980, soon after the completion of the cardiac wing, disaster struck. One of the walkways collapsed entirely. An investigation was commenced, and thirteen major structural faults were uncovered. Another problem concerned the water tanks located on the top floor. Their support was adequate as long as they were empty; if filled they would have collapsed. The building's shortfalls were a serious issue, as the cardiologists and radiologists had already moved into the new building and had started work there. The hospital administration asked for a list of all the people entering the building each morning. When we asked why we were told that they needed to know how many people were in the building if it collapsed!

The remedial building works were approved in April 1983 at a cost of £5 million, a figure later revised to £8 million. The final remedial works were authorized in January 1984 at a total cost of £13.4 million.

It was not until September 1987 that the wing was completed, and it became operational in January 1988. Fortunately the architects' and construction engineers' insurers covered the cost of the remedial work.

Prime Minister Margaret Thatcher officially opened the building in April 1988. It was an occasion of celebration, but incompetence had condemned us to additional years struggling to treat children in inadequate facilities.

19
MY BOOKS, 1979–1989

I used to play tennis regularly at Parliament Hill Fields. As Olga did not always feel like joining me she suggested that I ask a man we had spotted on a tennis court near by. We duly fixed a game for the following weekend, and from then on for several years the two of us played regularly at 8 a.m. every Sunday morning for an hour, first at Parliament Hill Fields, later at Highbury Fields.

One day Roger – we knew one another only by first names – arrived looking haggard with bags under his eyes. He said he would not give me a good game as he had got home very late the previous night from a party. He had been at the home of Donald Ross, a famous adult heart surgeon. It turned out that my tennis partner was Roger Farrand, managing director of Academic Press, a well-established publishing house, and he had gone to the gathering to try to persuade Ross to write a book on heart surgery. Until that day, although Roger and I had known one another for several years, I had no idea what he did for a living. He told me that Ross had said he was too old to embark on a new book and suggested Jarda Stark instead. Knowing that my first name was Jarda, Roger asked my surname. When I confirmed that it was Stark he immediately offered me a contract to write a cardiac surgery book. It was another example how different things were in Britain compared with my homeland. In Czechoslovakia if you sat on a train within half an hour your neighbours in the compartment would know what you did, how old your grandmother was and everything about you. In Britain if you wanted to retain some privacy this was respected.

So this was the beginning of my writing career. The idea grew on me more and more as I explored it with my colleague Marc de Leval, whom I thought would make a good co-editor. We discussed it also with Michael Courtney, a medical illustrator who used to work in the London Zoo as a technician anaesthetizing animals such as lions and cobras. He had previously prepared some illustrations for me when I was contributing to someone else's book, and he willingly agreed to cooperate on ours. Marc and I decided to write the major part of the book ourselves, but we wanted to involve experts from the UK, the USA and Australia.

To achieve uniformity in the style of illustration it was agreed that the outside contributors would provide us with sketches and that we would then work on the final versions with Michael. He started coming into the theatre, and sometimes we obtained pig hearts and undertook surgery in our office so that he could observe and make sketches. It took a long time, was a labour of love and hard work. The difficulties with the text were more to do with our co-authors who were often unhappy about our editorial interventions, but I remained firm on this.

Meanwhile Roger did not approve of the positioning of the illustrations. I did not want to have separate captions under the illustrations but make them an integral part of the text. Figure numbers would be indicated in bold, while the actual illustrations would be placed as close as possible to the related text. In the end Roger relented, and it was with some satisfaction that we noted that the first reviews mentioned the helpful placement of the illustrations as one of the most exceptional features of the book. The other positive comment was about the uniformity of the illustrations, which were presented from the perspective of the surgeon and not in the usual anatomical position employed so often in other publications.

The book was published in 1983, four years after we embarked on the project. Dwight McGoon wrote a very complimentary foreword. The reviews were very positive, and over the years it became known as *the* book of surgery for congenital heart defects. One of the best endorsements came years later via my friend Fernando Lucchese in Porto Alegre, Brazil. He told me that he had received a call from one of his former trainees who was working in a small hospital in Matto Grosso, miles from anywhere. They had admitted a newborn baby with transposition of the great arteries, and he had never operated on this before. Fernando asked if he had my book and told him to take it to theatre and to follow the pictures and the accompanying text. A very relieved surgeon phoned him back the next day saying that it had all gone well and the the baby had survived.

We eventually produced two more editions in 1993 and 2006. A second book, *Reoperations in Cardiac Surgery*, published in 1989, was instigated by my colleague Gerald Graham, a cardiologist at Great Ormond Street in charge of our team of perfusionists. He had an association with Springer Publications, and he thought it would be a good project. I agreed but thought that reoperations for congenital heart defects would be too limited a subject, so I decided to include adult cardiac surgery as well. As this was not my field I required a co-editor. I felt Al Pacifico from Birmingham, Alabama, would be the ideal candidate. He was an extremely competent congenital heart surgeon who also had considerable experience of working on valves and coronaries and undertaking cardiac operations on adults. He was happy to be involved, so it was settled. Michael Courtney agreed to illustrate the book, so we selected our contributors and started work.

One problem soon manifested itself. Al was happy to write his own chapters, but he was really not interested in the more general editorial work. It was left to me, despite the fact that my experience in adult cardiac surgery was merely academic. We were progressing well, but I was having problems with one of the authors, Dr Stanley Crawford from Texas, an undisputed king of surgery of aortic aneurysms who had written many works on the subject. He appointed two co-authors who, I suspected, merely rehashed one of his chapters from an earlier book. The sketches he provided were from the usual anatomical perspective, not as viewed by a working surgeon. I returned the chapter with my suggestions, but it came back more or less unchanged. I returned it once more, and after some weeks it arrived back in the form requested.

After the book was published in 1989 I received a cordial letter from Dr Crawford. 'Dear Dr Stark, this was the first time that a chapter of mine has been returned to me three times. But after viewing the book I have to agree with you. You were absolutely right. Congratulations!' I was delighted.

20
FURTHER TRIPS AND LECTURES, 1983–1985

I presented a paper and chaired a session on paediatric cardiology in Madrid in 1983 and participated at a meeting of the European Cardiac Surgeons' Club held in Hanover. The same year I was invited to a meeting in Erice, Sicily, where a number of prominent cardiac surgeons, including John Kirklin, attended. Several places such as Belgrade and Bordeaux were a delight to revisit soon after, while that September I had an opportunity to travel to Rio for the World Congress of the International Society for Cardiovascular Surgery. It was good to see all my friends again, including Paulo, a former resident at Great Ormond Street. Rio was considered at that time a highly dangerous city. We were warned that occasionally a person would be kidnapped, waking up the following morning with a large scar where a kidney had been removed for transplantation. During the Congress my Belgian friend Charles Chalant's female anaesthetist was mugged in front of the international hotel where we were staying.

I participated in London at a postgraduate symposium on the use of valves. They were used infrequently in children, and our budget allocation was for five a year. One year we had many more children requiring valve replacements. A request for extra money was turned down by the Department of Health, so I had to think of an alternative strategy. Bob Shenolikar, an Indian thoracic surgeon, was head of supplies at the Department of Health, and he enjoyed attending the clinical seminars at which we discussed indications for operations. We eventually gave him an honorary consultant contract in our department. I decided to write to him officially to explain our difficulty and suggested that we ask the parents of the children who needed artificial valves to raise the money themselves. I knew that this would be politically unacceptable, and I was right. A week later I had a reply saying that the Department of Health had allocated an extra £20,000 for the purchase of valves.

In October 1983 I was invited to the Spanish Society for Cardiovascular Surgery in Granada, and Olga accompanied me. We were told that Muslim architecture had reached its peak there. It was indeed remarkable, and Olga and I had a wonderful time visiting the Alhambra, including the Patio de los Leones, and the Generalife, the summer palace of the kings of Granada famed for its terraced gardens. We also had a chance to visit the cathedral. The first evening we went to see flamenco dancing, which was extremely impressive. The performance finished at about midnight, and after that the annual society dinner was held in an old monastery. Olga and I were sitting at the top table, and at about 2.30 a.m. Pedro Sanchez, secretary of the society, stood up and started reading his annual report in a monotone. He went on and on; it was like a scene in a Buñuel movie. At about 4 a.m. Olga and I decided we had enough and sneaked out. I was aware that the next morning I was supposed to participate at a panel on congenital heart surgery at 9 a.m. When I arrived there was one other lecturer at the door, which was still locked. At 9.20 the projectionist arrived and unlocked it. By 9.45 five out of the eight members of the panel had arrived and just a few participants. The chairman decided to start the session at 10 a.m. All the panellists were there but just nine people in the audience. I was appalled. They had invited top paediatric cardiac surgeons from all over Europe and two from the USA, whose air fares and hotels had been paid for, and this was the result. But one must hand it to the Spaniards: they do enjoy life.

In December I travelled to Taiwan to the Asia Pacific meeting. Dr Chiu was a former fellow at Great Ormond Street, and he looked after me during my stay. A visit to the National Museum was one of the highlights, as it was considered one of the wonders of the world. It is rumoured that when Chiang Kai-shek left mainland China he arrived with a train full of treasures now exhibited in Taipei. I spent the whole afternoon in the museum, as it was such an amazing collection. Dr Chiu also took me on a trip around the island, which I enjoyed greatly, as I found the Chinese friendly and it was a fascinating place to visit.

In 1984 I attended a meeting of the Scandinavian Society of Cardiothoracic Surgery in Oslo. Before I was presented with my honorary membership, Ilmo Louhimo, the chief paediatric cardiac surgeon from Helsinki, introduced me in verse:

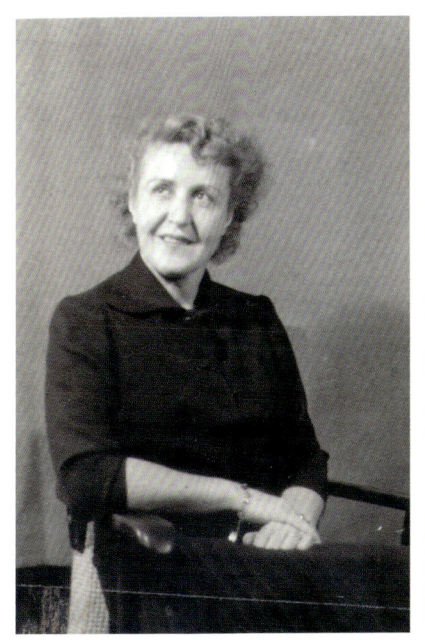

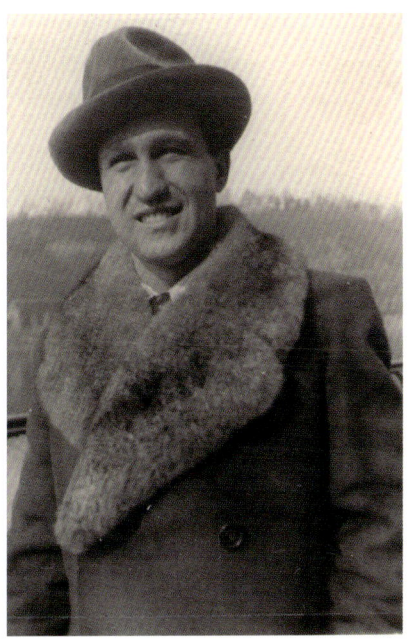

Above: My mother, Jiřina Starková (1911–1992), and my father, Jaroslav Stark (1907–1994), in 1939

Below: With my paternal grandfather, Jaroslav, at six months

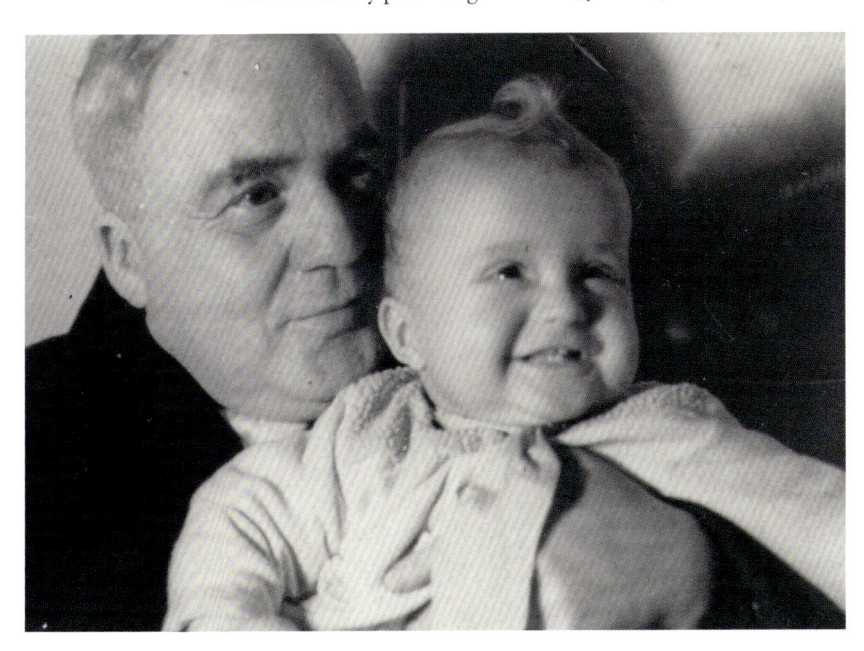

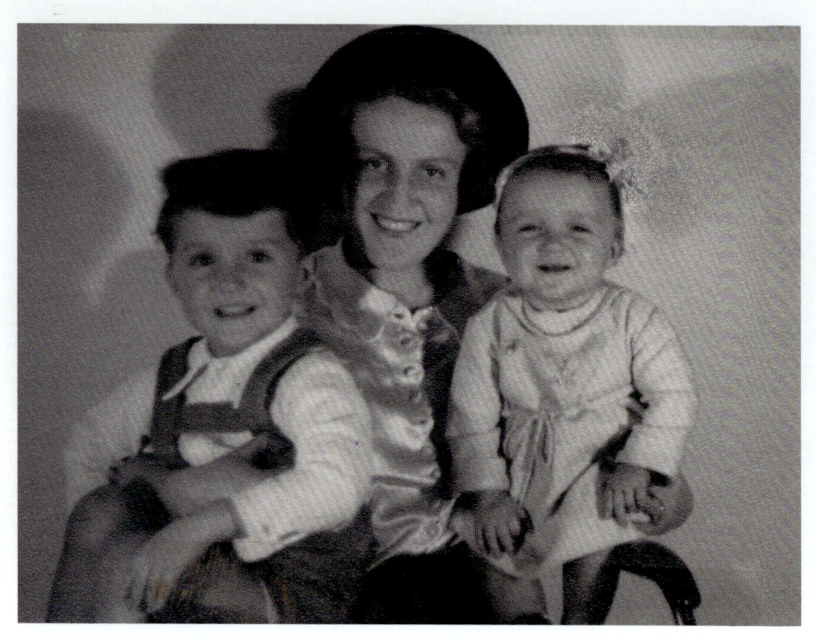

Above: In 1937, aged three, with my mother and six-month-old sister, Jiřina, who was born in 1937

Below: On my rocking-horse, 1938

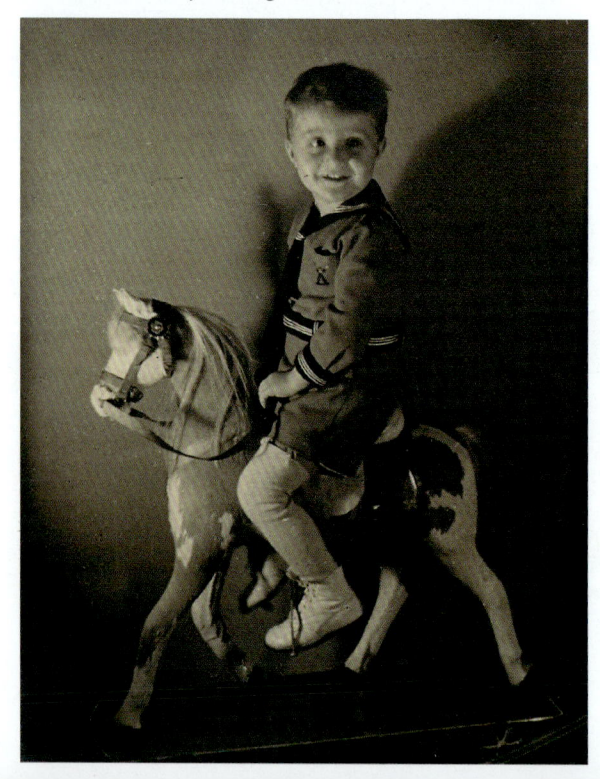

Right: Me skiing in Radhošt in 1940; little did I know then that I would still be skiing in the Alps fifty years later.

Below: The family summer-house in the village of Senohraby, 30 kilometres south-east of Prague, as it is today; it was built by my father in 1939.

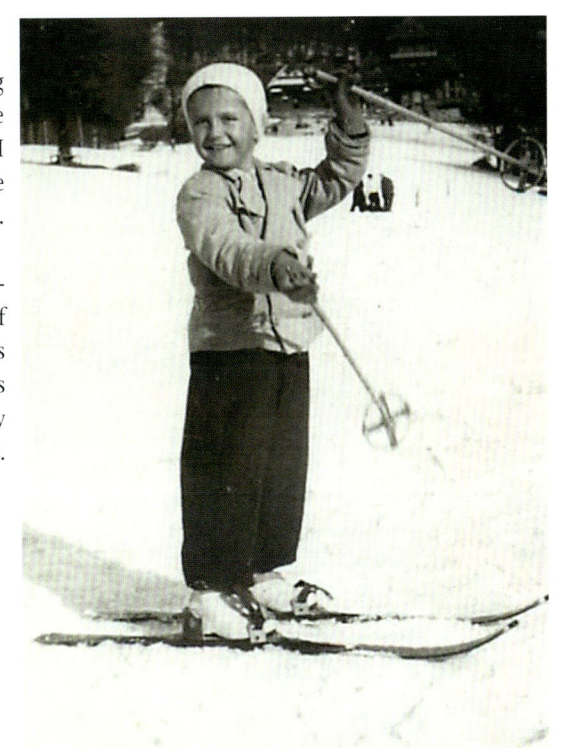

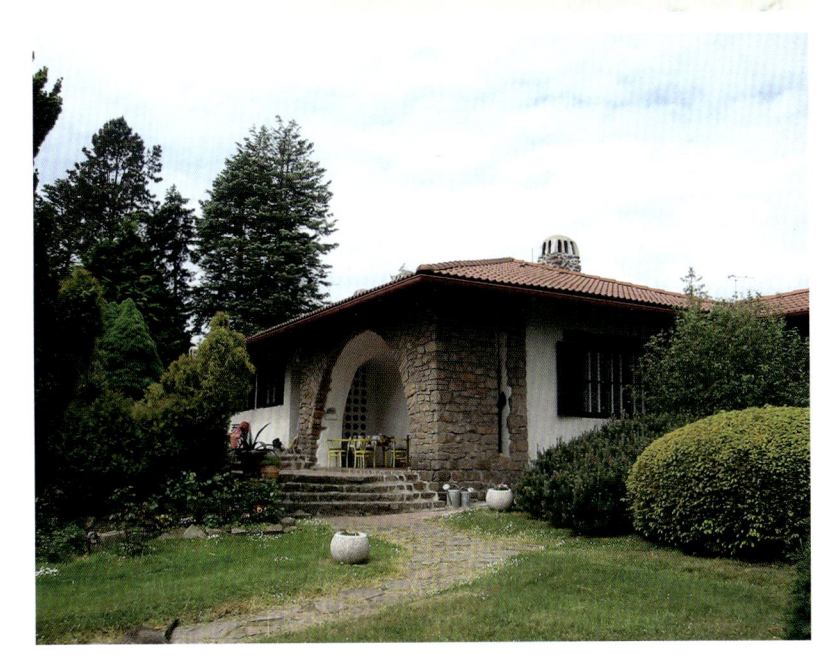

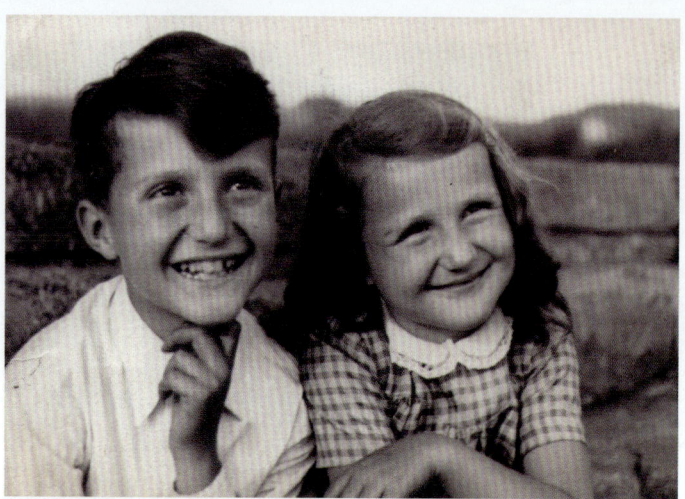

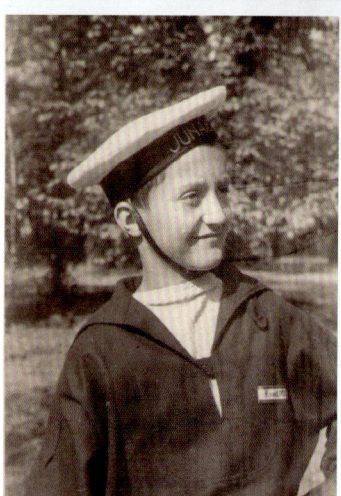

Top: With Jiřina in Senohraby, 1941

Left: As a Sea Scout, 1947

Below: With my father in Senohraby, 1955

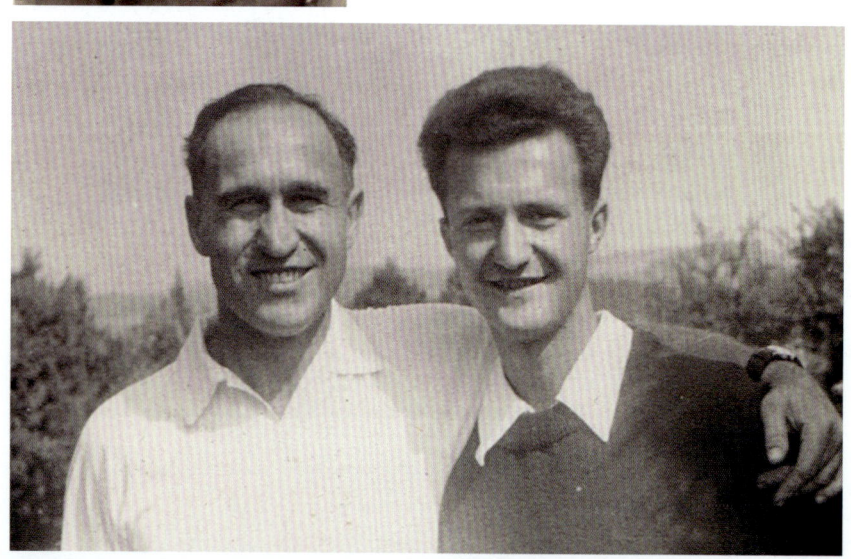

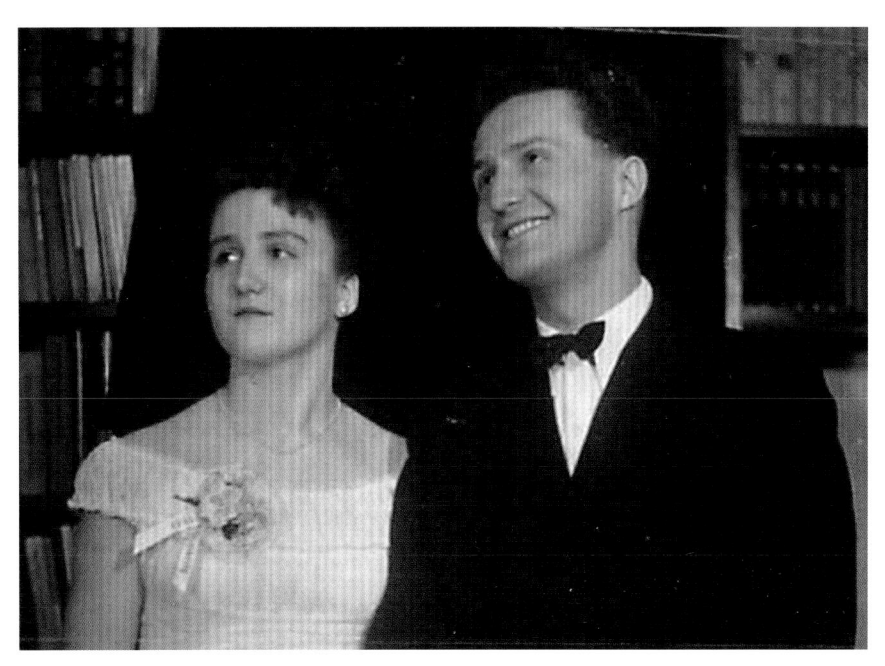

Above: With Jiřina before her secondary-school ball, *c.* 1953

Below: Olga (née Slugová) after her graduation ceremony, 1958

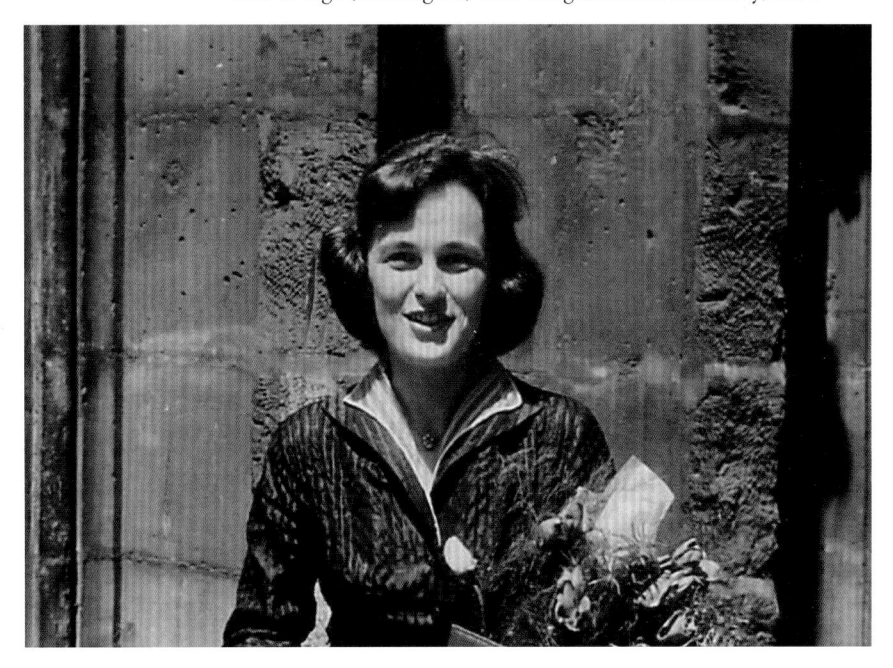

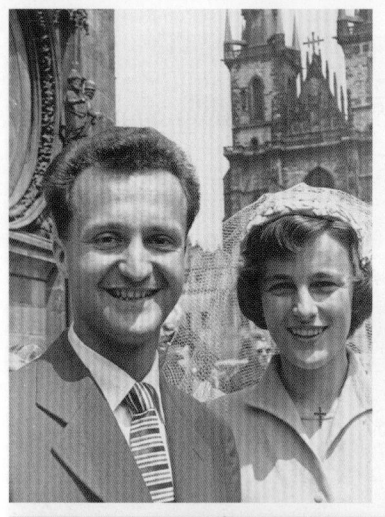

Left and below (middle): Olga and I are married in Prague, 1959

Bottom: Our wedding day, 1959; me with Olga along with Saša Kučera, my best friend, parody Stalin's monument (seen in the distance just to my left). If we had been caught we could have received jail sentences of up to ten years.

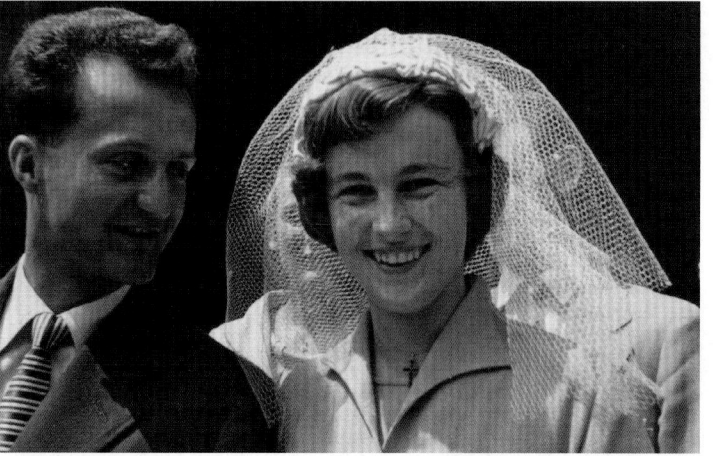

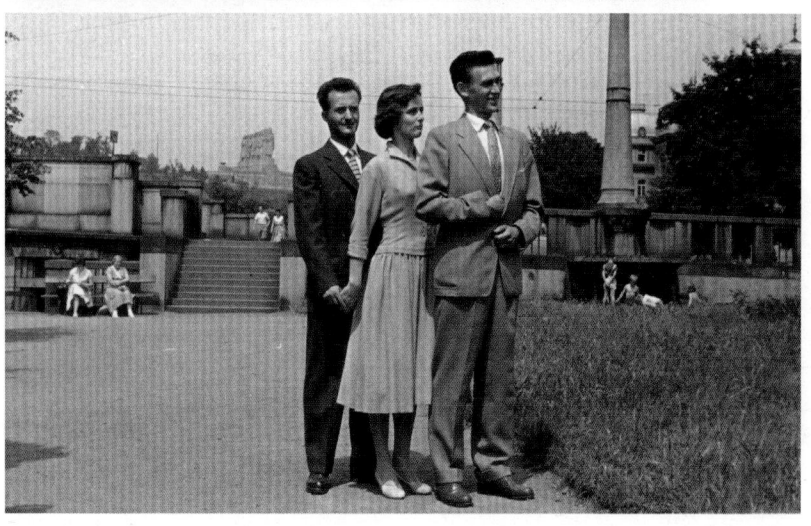

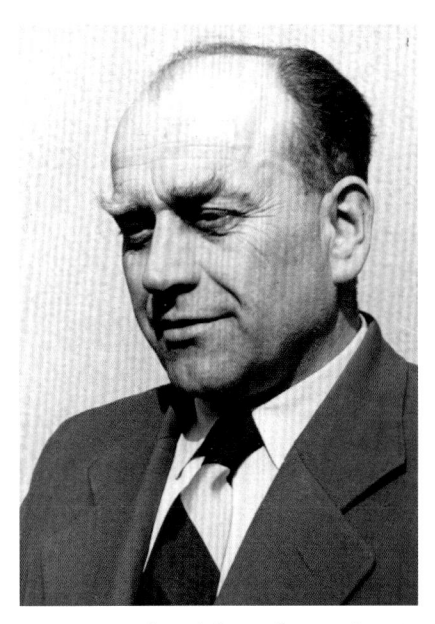

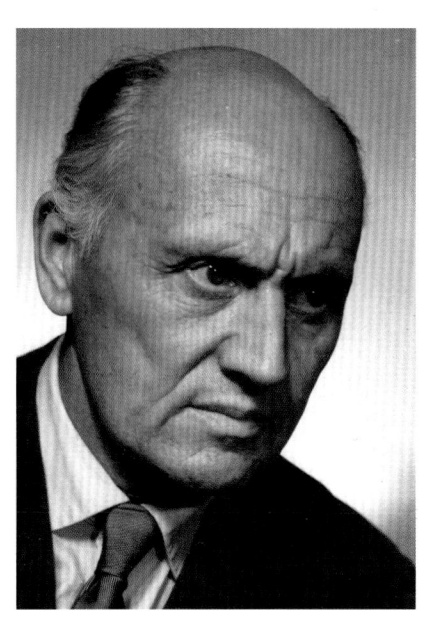

Above left: My first teacher, Dr Jaroslav Kudr, in Rychnov nad Kněžňou, Czechoslovakia,1962
Above right: Professor Václav Kafka, head of the Department of Paediatric Surgery, University Hospital, Prague, 1964

Below left: David Waterson, my consultant at Great Ormond Street,1969
Below right: Iain Aberdeen, the other consultant at Great Ormond Street, late 1960s

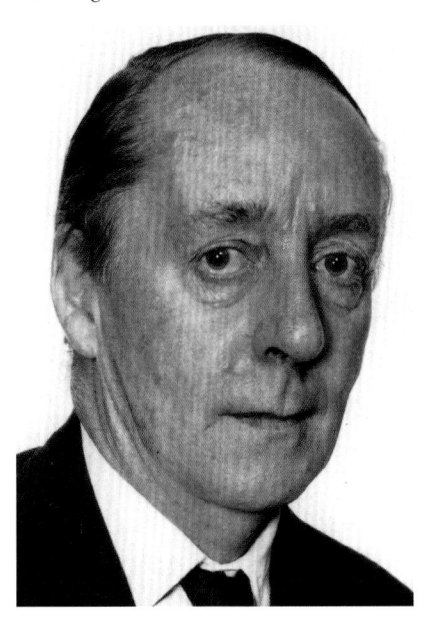

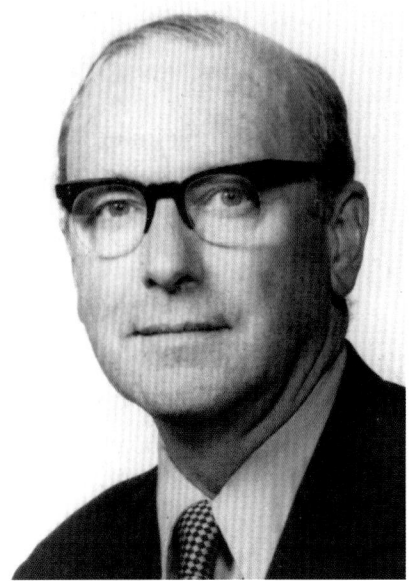

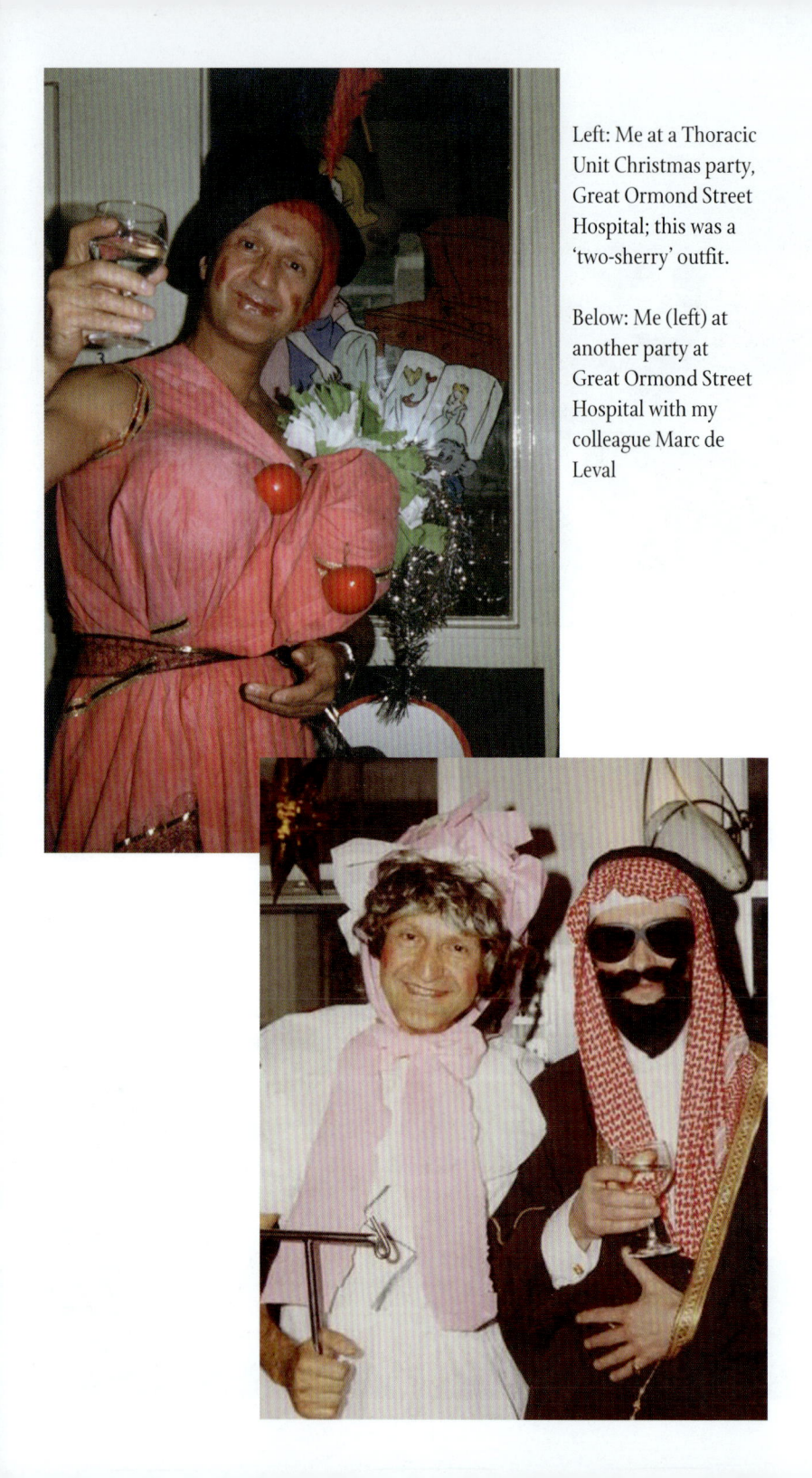

Left: Me at a Thoracic Unit Christmas party, Great Ormond Street Hospital; this was a 'two-sherry' outfit.

Below: Me (left) at another party at Great Ormond Street Hospital with my colleague Marc de Leval

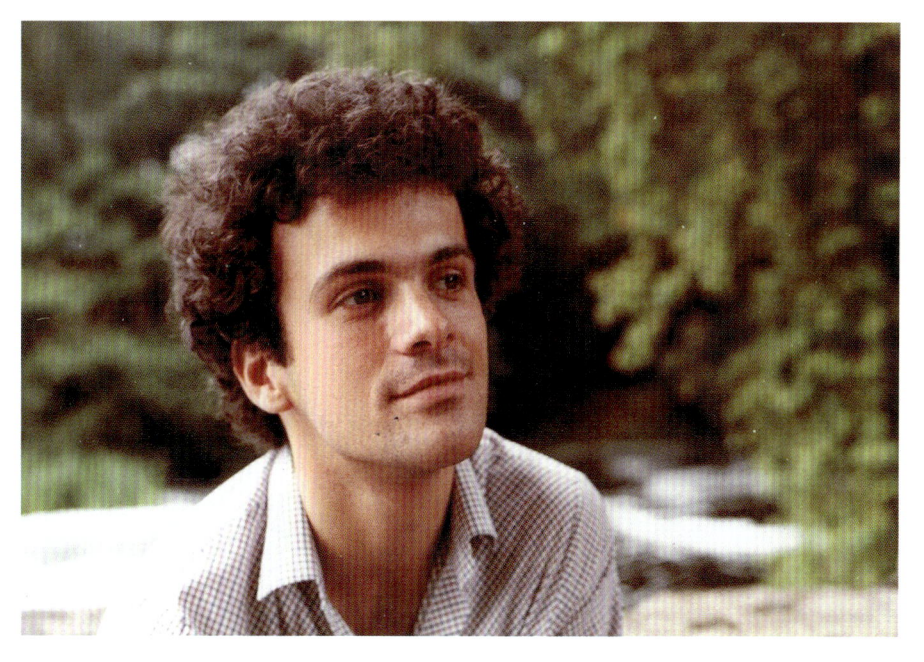

Above: My son Jaroslav, 1979; he went up to Cambridge University in 1978.

Below: The three Jaroslavs – my son, my father and me – Austria, 1983

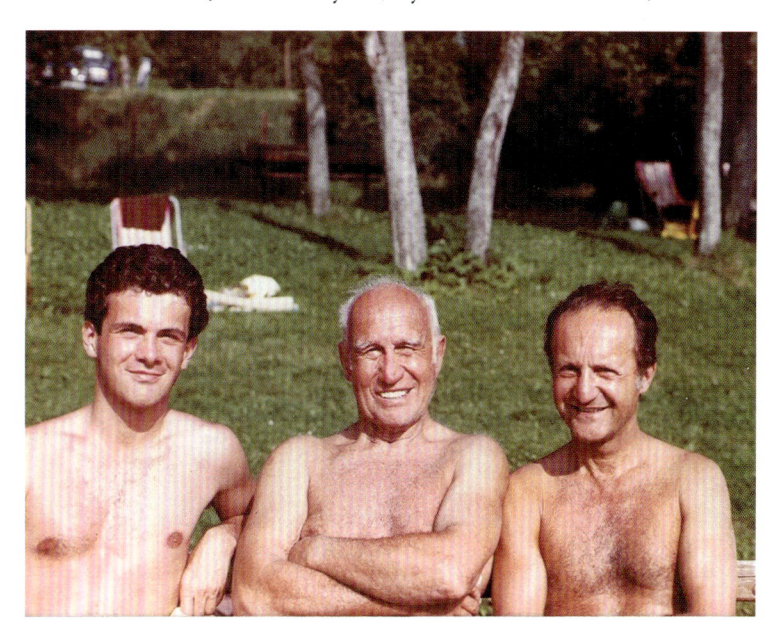

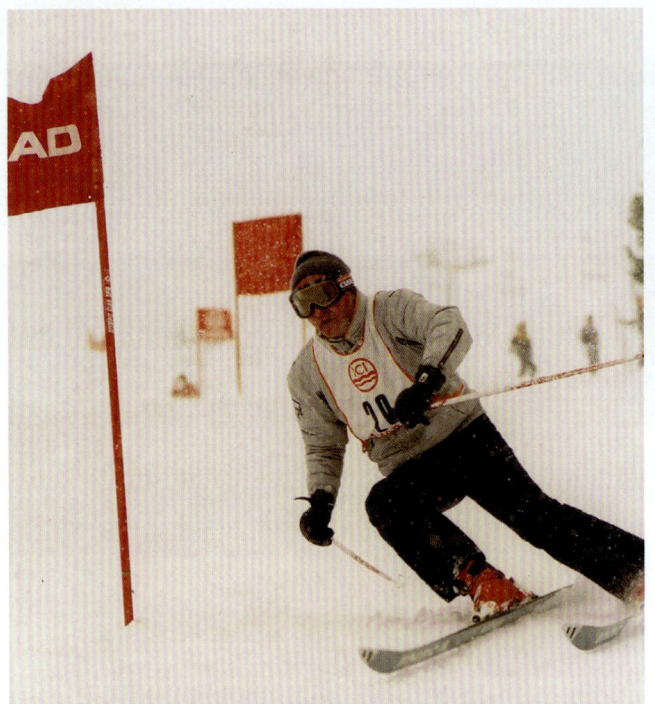

Left: Me negotiating the giant slalom during the annual 'Cardiac' skiing meeting in Courcheval, 1986

Below: With Bill Williams in Toronto, late 1980s

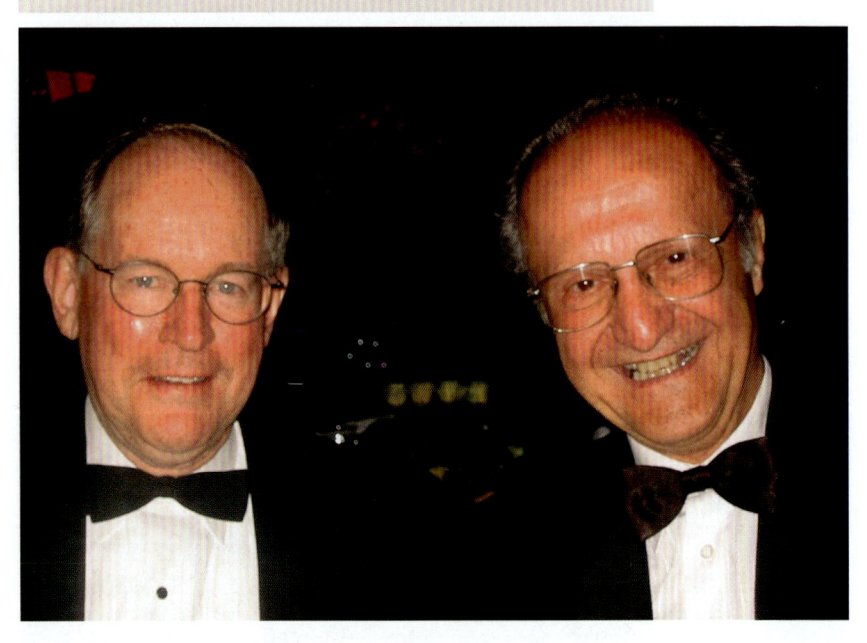

Right: Jaroslav and Kate (née Hardy) on their wedding day, 30 May 1987, at Islington Register Office, London

Below: The wedding reception at Anson Road, Tufnell Park, London

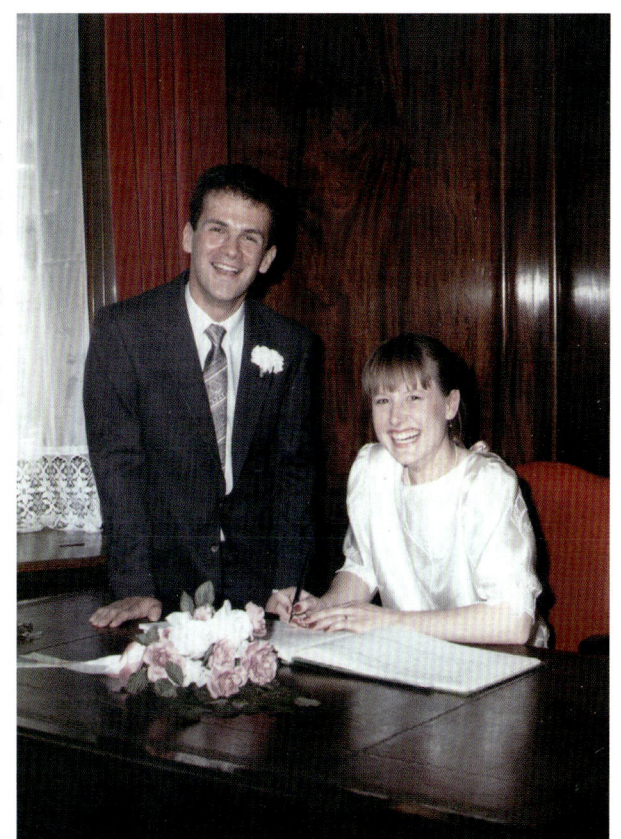

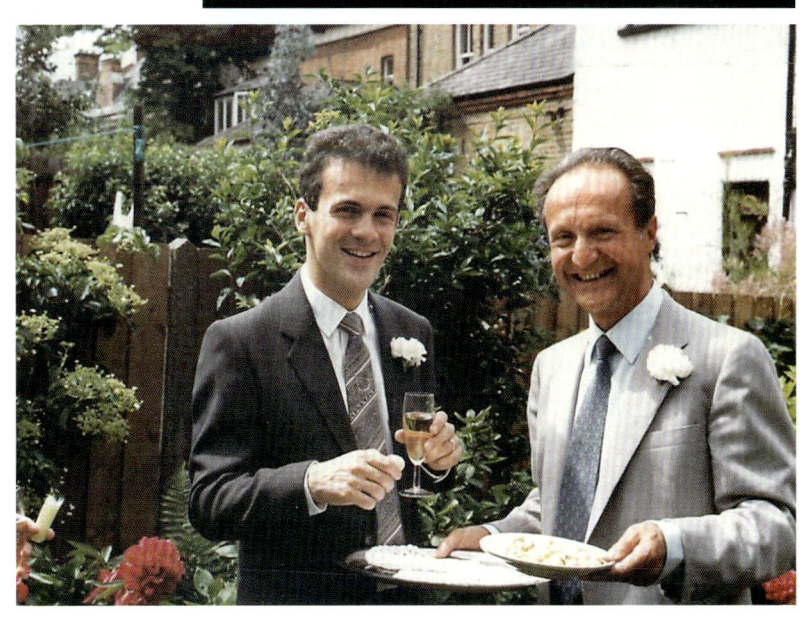

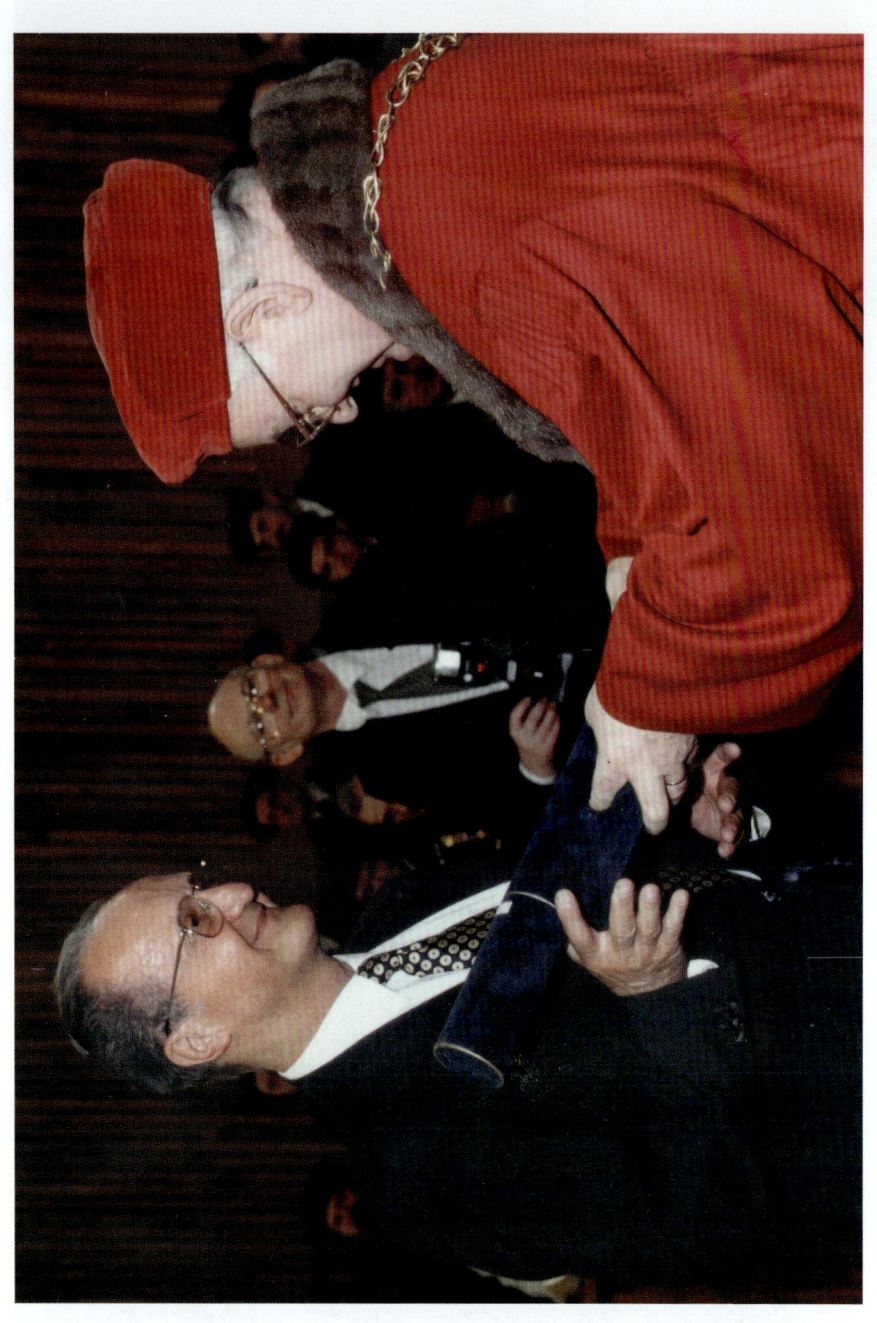

Receiving the gold medal at Charles University, Prague,
on the occasion of the institution's 650th anniversary, 1998

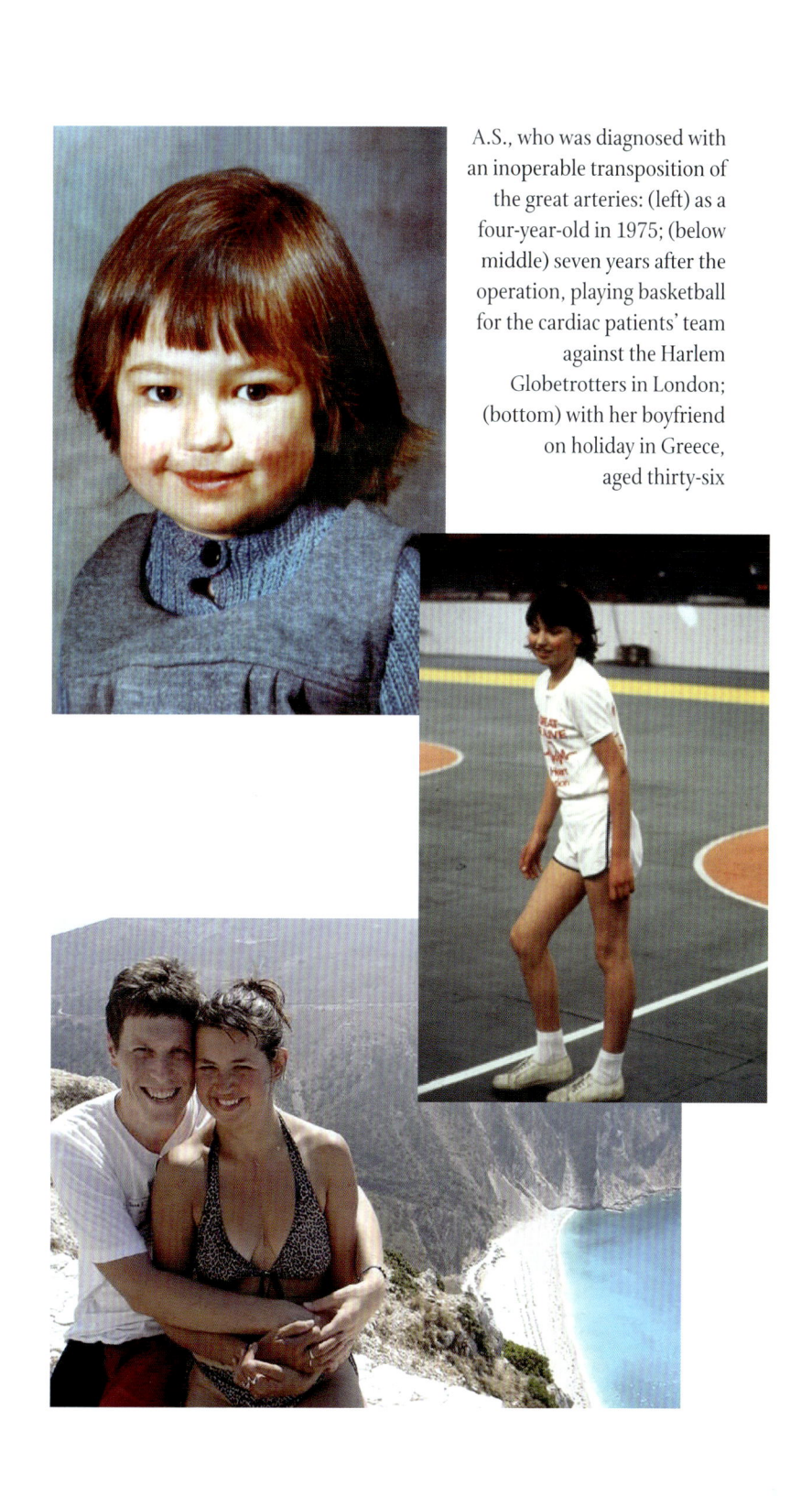

A.S., who was diagnosed with an inoperable transposition of the great arteries: (left) as a four-year-old in 1975; (below middle) seven years after the operation, playing basketball for the cardiac patients' team against the Harlem Globetrotters in London; (bottom) with her boyfriend on holiday in Greece, aged thirty-six

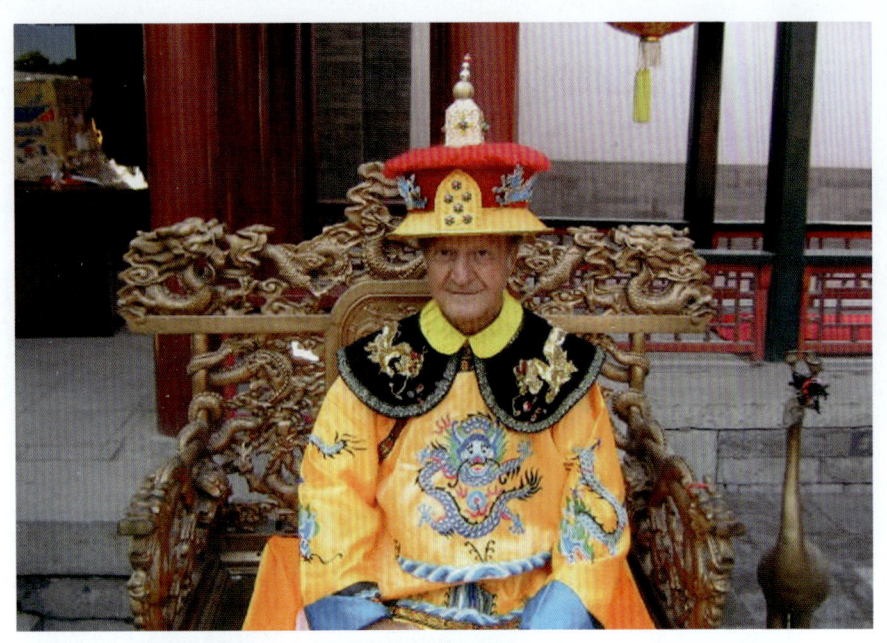

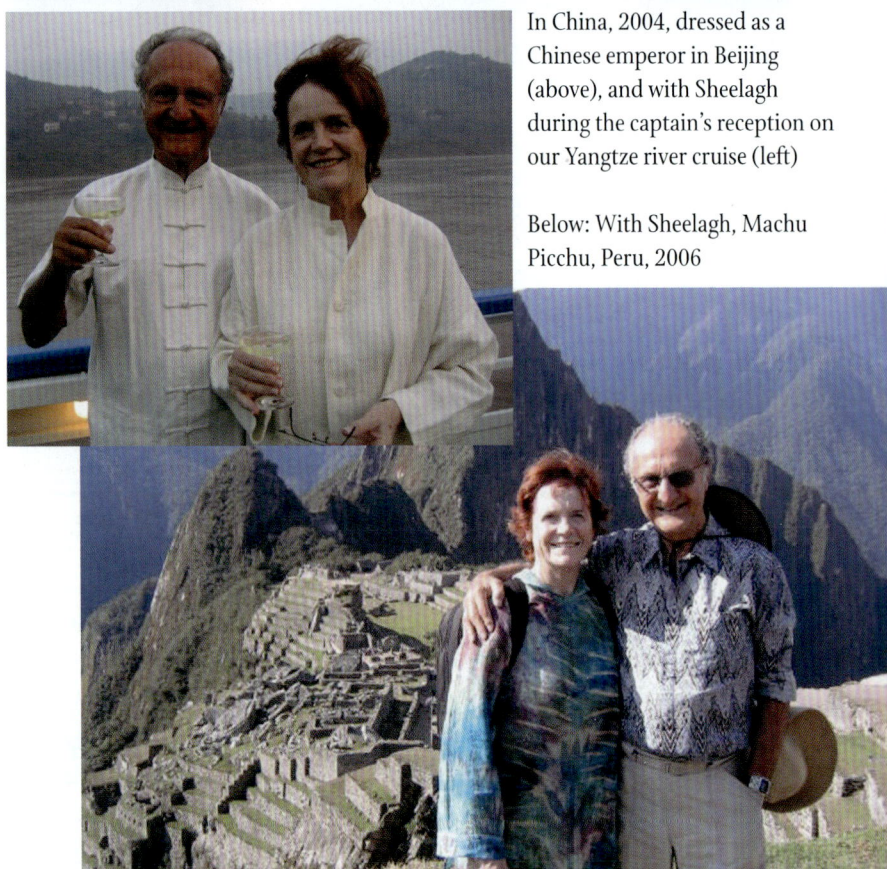

In China, 2004, dressed as a Chinese emperor in Beijing (above), and with Sheelagh during the captain's reception on our Yangtze river cruise (left)

Below: With Sheelagh, Machu Picchu, Peru, 2006

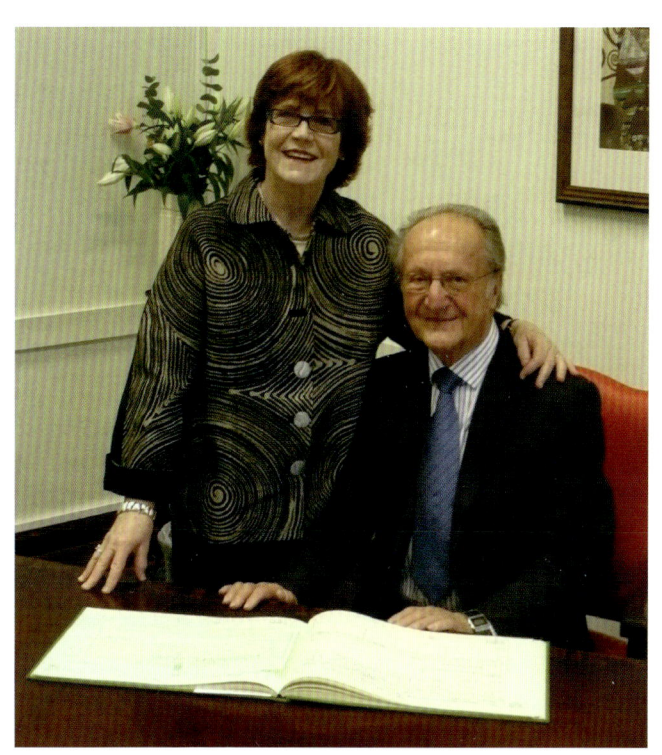

Above: Sheelagh and I are married on 1 February 2011 at Islington Register Office

Right: Grandson Daniel with his mother Kate

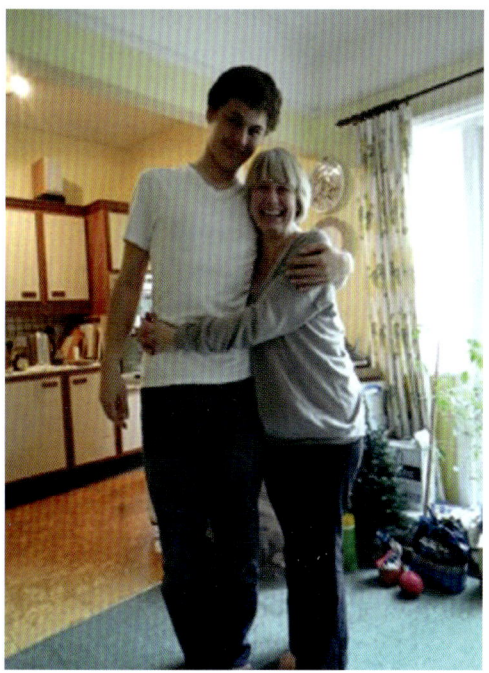

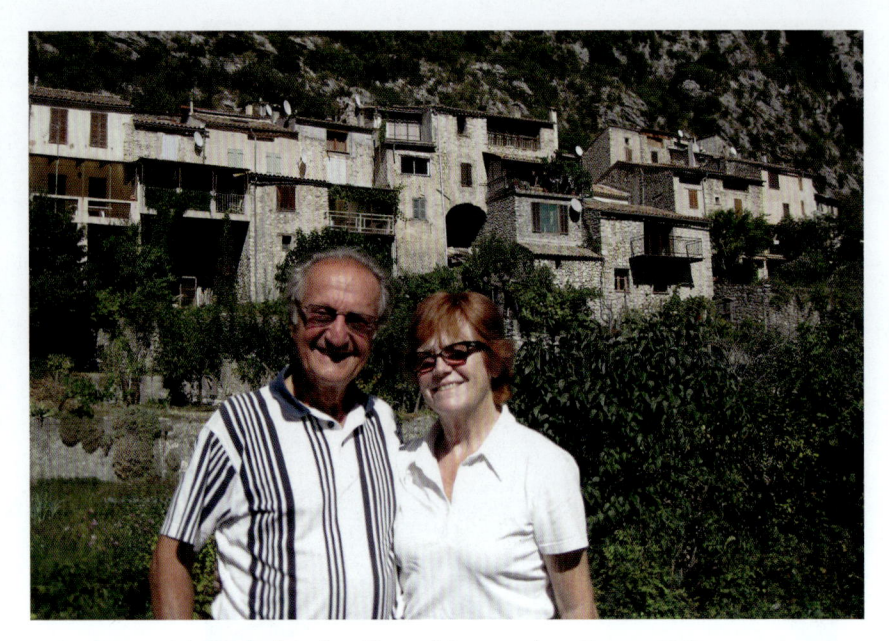

Above: With Sheelagh in the village of Gars, southern France, 2013

Below: In November 2014 I received a silver medal from Charles University, Prague, and a gold medal from the Medical School. The ceremony was held in the old Gothic hall in the Karolinum, where I had been presented with my medical degree in 1958.

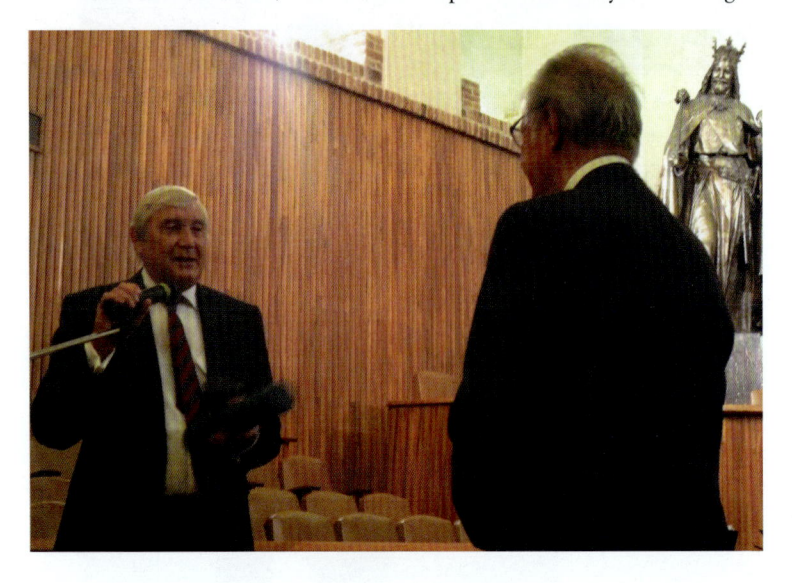

> To this our meeting
> His personal mark
> Again now has given
> Our guest Jarda Stark.
> I hope you can see him
> Although it is dark
> His smile over there
> Is the smile of a shark.
> Or maybe he looks like a dangerous wolf
> As I could not fix him
> His session of golf.
> I tell you that also
> My eyes have a tear;
> I blame for it Jarda
> As Olga isn't here.

The second verse from Ilmo came the next day before my lecture:

> On whom we now set spotlight's beam
> He is a man of skiing team.
> The leading guest he has been twice
> He wrote a book quite new and nice.
> To the very top he made his way
> By treating babies' TGA.
> Quite far from home this man has gone
> First learning skills of Waterston
> And later just to save his neck;
> By now you know he is a Czech.
> He certainly has made his mark
> I am speaking of Jaroslav Stark.

During the presidential dinner I was sitting with Gudmund Semb, my friend from the Cardiac Surgeons' Club. While the port was being served I asked whether I would be asked to speak. He told me not to worry. Walter Lillihei, one of the grandees of cardiac surgery, an American with Scandinavian ancestors, was in attendance. He would be asked to speak, Gudmund assured me. So I had a second glass of port. Two minutes later the master of ceremonies tapped me on the shoulder and said, 'Would you mind saying a few words? I can give you five minutes.' It was likely to be a very awkward five minutes. Fortunately Matthias Paneth from the Brompton Hospital was in the audience. He used to enjoy putting me down, so I based my brief speech on making fun of him by way of retaliation. It went down very well. Afterwards when we strolled into an adjacent room he came up behind me, tapping me on the shoulder, saying, 'Jarda, fifteen all!' During the dancing that followed I was sitting at the top table, next to Inge Rygg's second wife. Inge was the chief surgeon from Copenhagen, the inventor of the Rygg's oxygenator, while his wife had a reputation for mischief. When Matthias came up and asked her to dance, she said loudly, 'Is that you, Dr Paneth? I didn't recognize you with your clothes on.' He had spent a few days before the meeting with Inge and his wife in their summer cottage and in their sauna. Her comment was heard all over the dance floor and resulted in general mirth.

Later in the year I chaired a session at the American College of Cardiology meeting in Dallas, went to the International Congress of the European Society of Cardiac Surgery in Madrid and to an international symposium on the double inlet ventricle in Bergamo.

The British Heart Foundation gave us money for the chair of paediatric cardiology. I was very much hoping that we would appoint Mike Tynan, who was by this time a consultant cardiologist in Newcastle. Mike was a brilliant guy and an excellent cardiologist who was ready to learn new skills. Unfortunately he was also very unorthodox – turning up at the hospital in country boots and not respecting the authority of certain senior consultants, for example – so he was vetoed by members of the appointment committee. I vetoed other candidates, so we found ourselves in a stalemate. Some months later the post was readvertised, and Fergus Macartney was appointed. Unfortunately Mike Tynan took against me, even though he was aware that I had supported him to the hilt, and he never forgave me. After that our relationship went downhill, even though he was eventually appointed professor at Guy's Hospital.

That November I was invited to Saudi Arabia and Kuwait. The airport in Riyadh was very modern with many stunning water features. The hotel was a five-star one with restrictions on the presence of women at the pool, despite the intense heat. Next day Olga and I were taken for a tour of the city, including the main square where every Friday punishments were meted out. Burglars got their hands chopped off, and more serious crimes were punished by beheading. At the end of the day all the chopped-off body parts were cleared away and the square returned to its normal function for the rest of the week. A Scottish couple, who had lived and worked in Riyadh for two years, told us that they had never gone to watch the punishments. I could understand why.

The Falcons market and the gold souk were less gruelling. We also went to see the palaces. Some years earlier one of the Saudi princes had visited the USA and admired the White House. On his return he asked his architects to build him a larger version, so the city has its own White House. In the hospital they had three swimming-pools – one for men, one for women and another for children. I met a nurse who had been at Great Ormond Street who told me that many things in everyday life were frustrating to her as a woman working out there and that sometimes she found it almost impossible to stick to the letter of the law. For instance, it was illegal for women to drive a vehicle, and during the night she could not be in a car with a man who was not her husband; traffic police would actually ask to see a marriage certificate.

During the meeting I was told a joke. An orthopaedic surgeon operated on a Saudi prince. Afterwards the prince asked him what he would like as a thank-you present. The doctor did not want anything, but after some arm-twisting he requested a set of golf clubs. Nothing appeared for three months, but after nine months he received a cable. 'Set of golf clubs almost complete. Sorry, not all of them have a swimming-pool.'

The meeting started with the mullah reciting verses from the Koran. As there were so many Western visitors it surprised me that he stressed the punishment awaiting unbelievers. I presented two papers at the meeting. The evening reception was at the US ambassador's house, which was exceptionally beautiful and which had a large swimming-pool. Everybody was looking forward to a drink, but nothing alcoholic was served – apparently at the express instigation of the head of Riyadh's cardiac surgery unit, Dr Al-Faghi. Another dinner – dry again – was hosted in Dr Al-Faghi's house. He had trained in the USA and at the Brompton Hospital, but I noted that his wife did not appear at all. At the end of the evening Olga and the wives were invited to visit her in her quarters. I talked to Dr Al-Faghi's brother, a urologist, who told me that the Saudis sent women to university but that when they finished their studies they were not allowed to further their education abroad unless one of their male relatives accompanied them.

When we were in Saudi Arabia we were unable to go to Kuwait, as there was political unrest, so Olga and I decided to pay a short visit to Egypt and flew to Cairo. Immediately after arriving we were marched to the bank where we had to change $150 at the official rate, although we were allowed to change the rest of our money at a more favourable tourist rate. After some brief sightseeing in Cairo we flew to Luxor where we visited the main temple. At the site we saw a person with leprosy for the first time – an unsettling experience.

We visited the temple in Karnak with its impressive Hypostyle Hall with 134 enormous columns; it was said that it had been calculated that a hundred people could stand on the top of just one of them. We were perplexed as to how they had managed to get these from Aswan to Karnak and erect them. The local guides offered their services on every corner, which we found intrusive, so we spoke to them in Czech and pretended that we did not understand a word of English.

The following day we headed for the local ferry that took us across the Nile. On the other side we were surrounded by an army of mule handlers, taxi drivers and guides. After a while we started haggling and eventually got a good price for a drive to the Valley of the Kings. Unfortunately our taxi driver was from the other side of the river so was regarded as 'illegal'. There was much shouting, and the driver at the front of the queue called the tourist police. We eventually left in another taxi with a policeman in the front seat. The Valley of the Kings was amazing. In front of the tomb of Ramesses II was a statue they thought had been about 17 metres tall and weighing over 1,000 tonnes. How they had transported it along the Nile was anyone's guess. The tomb of Tutankhamen was particularly impressive, even though most of its contents had been moved to the museum in Cairo. One can only marvel at how surprised and astonished Howard Carter must have been when he discovered the tomb intact, containing four gold shrines, one inside the other, and a stone sarcophagus with three coffins. The one that contained the body of the pharaoh was made of pure gold and weighed 1,128 kilograms.

When at the mortuary of the huge Temple of Hatshepsut we were told that one was not allowed to take pictures with flash, but a small quantity of 'baksheesh' did the trick, and the guard made sure that no one saw me snapping away. The taxi driver suggested that we walk across the mountain to the Valley of the Queens. This took about two hours, and he told us that he would meet us there. It sounded like a good idea, so off we went. We started climbing, but soon the local guides spotted us and desperately tried to catch up with us to offer their services. We were good walkers, so it took some time for them to catch up. When they did and we categorically refused to use them they were bitterly disappointed. Nevertheless the visit to the valleys was a memorable experience. The paintings on the walls of the tombs were remarkable, and the setting was fabulous.

The next day we crossed the Nile where our taxi driver from the previous day was waiting for us, and we discussed what we wanted to see. He took us to a kiosk to buy tickets, where we got two student ones as a special deal, and we drove to the Valley of the Nobles. Most of the paintings on the walls did not look especially old, as they were so well preserved, but they had been there for millennia. In Deir el-Medina was a tomb of Senudjen, a servant in the Place of Truth. The paintings on the walls of his tomb were especially exquisite.

On the last day of our holidays we took a bus to the airport for a flight to Cairo, where we spent considerable time in the vast archaeological museum. The excavations from Tutankhamen's tomb were particularly breathtaking. After spending some five hours in the museum we were overwhelmed.

In the afternoon we took a taxi to the pyramids. The traffic was unbelievable, as drivers overtake on the left, right and centre, missing each other by centimetres. Our driver was highly experienced, but even so we had a few tense moments. When we arrived at the pyramids the sun was setting, so it provided us with wonderful light for photography. As usual, as soon as we got out of the taxi we were surrounded by hordes of guides and youngsters offering their services to tourists. We spent most of our time getting rid of them. The individual stone blocks from which the pyramids are constructed are approximately two and a half tonnes in weight. They are so well chiselled that they fit together without cement, and it is said that a razor blade could not be placed between them.

The next morning we took a taxi to the airport. Everything was totally disorganized, with endless officials checking the luggage, but it was all done rather superficially. We had a feeling that one could smuggle through a machine-gun. Then we had to change money, but everything was arranged in such a way that this was nigh on impossible. Yet one was not allowed to take Egyptian currency out of the country. In the end I talked to the manager of the local bank branch, and when threatened with an official complaint he arranged the monetary exchange.

In 1985 I lectured in Rome, Philadelphia, London and Kuwait. In Kuwait my friends told me that David Waterston and Dick Bonham Carter had been invited there a few years earlier. At the customs check at the airport they found a bottle of whisky in Bonham Carter's suitcase. David was quick to save the situation. He explained to the customs officer that his friend was an alcoholic and needed the whisky as medicine and he would have to let him through. It worked!

The European Cardiac Surgeons' Club meeting that year was held in Crans Montana in Switzerland, with an enjoyable dinner at Charlie Hahn's house near Lausanne.

In June I participated at the World Congress of Paediatric Cardiology in New York. Immediately after my return to London Olga and I had a frightening experience. I was tired and went to bed early and was woken up at about 2 a.m. by her screaming and banging on the inside of our bedroom door. I asked what was going on, and she told me a noise had woken her up. The door to the bedroom had opened and a man in a balaclava had walked in. At first she thought it was one of my bad jokes, but on seeing me in the bed next to her she realized it was an intruder. She felt her best form of defence was to scream loudly. This worked. 'Who can stand a hysterical woman?' she said. The man raced down the stairs to the ground floor and fled. Later we realized that he had got in through a small window in the kitchen. Police told us that there was a rapist operating in our area, so we never knew whether he was a thief or a rapist. As I had been away for more than a week he may have been observing our house and realized that Olga was on her own. Subsequently we had metal bars put up at the window as well as on the doors from the kitchen to the garden.

In New York I met a good friend from my Boy Scout days, Vojta Volavka. Vojta had married Jitka Horčičková, a Czech tennis champion and an excellent skier. After the Russian invasion they had packed their car and driven west to Germany. About a year later they moved from Munich to the

USA, first to New York and later to St Louis, where Vojta became professor of psychiatry at the university. Unfortunately their marriage did not work out, and Jitka left him for a good friend of his who was an anaesthetist. The legal proceedings left Vojta with very little money, and at the same time he faced a highly stressful medical court case. He had been involved in research into the electroencephalogram (EEG) response to treatment of drug users. This was conducted in a large enclosed unit on an island just off New York. One drug addict who developed Parkinson's disease accused Vojta, claiming that this was as a consequence of a drug he had prescribed. Vojta researched the literature not only in English but also in French, German and Russian and did not find a single article linking the drug with the onset of Parkinson's disease. However, his insurance company decided to settle out of court despite strong protests from Vojta. They said, 'You never know how the jury will react when they see this poor guy in dirty clothes on one side and an affluent doctor on the other.' It meant that in the insurance world nobody would insure Vojta, so he had to give up his private practice.

Vojta, however, was to remarry. One of his relatives sent him a package containing kitchen knives, asking Vojta to deliver them to Jana, a Czech girl living in California. She had decided to emigrate, so she packed two pairs of skis and asked for permission to travel to a competition in California. Surprisingly, permission was granted, and she managed to leave the country in July. Although she had a degree in chemistry, she was employed washing dishes in California. Vojta sent her the knives, and a couple of months later – on impulse – he wrote to her saying that he was going to ski at Christmas in Jackson Hole in Wyoming and asked if she would like to join him there. She said yes. He wrote back saying that a single room was $150 each and a double was $180. Which should he book? She suggested a double room and arrived in Jackson Hole just before Christmas when Vojta was out skiing. She sat in the bedroom feeling very nervous, not knowing what to expect, as she had never met him before. Eventually he came back, and it turned out well. They went for a cross-country outing with a group, as they were both physically very fit. After about 10 kilometres they took a break. The guide suggested a snack, but as Vojta had taken a bottle of whisky with him he took it out in front of the horrified guide and was warned that they wouldn't be able to keep up the pace. But when they got going again Vojta and Jana were so fast that the guide had difficulty keeping up with them.

After this they remained friends. Jana was still working in California and Vojta in New York, so they saw one another only occasionally. One day they were at the Metropolitan Museum and were sitting on a circular bench in the hall where Vojta was trying to persuade Jana to move in with him in his flat in New York. To persuade her he said, 'And I promise always to raise the loo seat when I go for a pee.' At which point an elderly lady sitting next to them on the bench said in perfect Czech, 'Why don't you marry him when he's asking so nicely?'

That year Olga and I purchased a small apartment in Val d'Isère, our favourite ski resort. Olga called it a glorified cupboard, as it was only 21 square metres, but it was fine. There was a sitting-room with a lovely view over the Solaise mountain, a favourite place of ours to ski. We had a couch there that opened out into a double bed. In the adjacent small cabin there would normally be three bunk beds, but as we had a false ceiling constructed for storage we had just a single bed there with drawers under the bed. There was a small well-equipped kitchen and a bathroom with a toilet. The resort had more then 250 kilometres of pistes, so, as far as I was concerned, it was paradise. Eventually we gave the apartment to Jaroslav and Kate when I could no longer ski because of my various joint replacements, but we enjoyed many holidays there.

21
ON SABBATICAL, 1986–1987

Fergus Macartney, a professor of cardiology at Great Ormond Street, took a sabbatical year in 1985. He was an academic, but I felt that I had worked hard since 1971 and that I deserved a sabbatical, too. So I applied. At first there was not much support for this, but then it was agreed that I would get six months' leave without pay. I think that shortly after this some of my colleagues on the medical committee realized that that their decision might set a bad precedent, since if any one of them applied for a sabbatical subsequently it would also have to be without pay. I was not especially worried about the financial side of things, as I could support myself with the money I received from lecturing, but in the end I was granted a six months' sabbatical on full pay.

A further reason for taking a sabbatical at this particular time was the many problems with the newly constructed cardiac wing. Many newly appointed staff, including another surgeon, were already in place, waiting patiently until the remedial work was completed, so I felt that my absence would not be a problem.

I planned to take the sabbatical in two stages, the first three months in the USA, then return to the UK and take the second three months in Europe. My idea was to visit some cardiac departments, but my priority during the second part of my sabbatical was to finish my second book, *Reoperations in Cardiac Surgery*. In 1986 I left for the USA. My first stop was Nashville, Tennessee. Harvey Bender, the chief of cardiac surgery, met me at the airport and took me to my hotel, a Holiday Inn. Originally the plan was that I would stay with Harvey and after that with the head of cardiology, but being in a hotel gave me far more freedom, so I was happy with this arrangement.

In Nashville they had a very good record for operating on infants with atrioventricular septal defect (AVSD), but, as I found was often the case, things were never as straightforward or successful as some of the department's literature suggested. They scheduled three babies with AVSD to be operated on during my stay. The first died on the table, the second was fine and the third was still on a ventilator five days later when I left the unit.

In terms of living accommodation, I was impressed by my hosts' huge houses, although some of the interior decoration seemed brash. Each house was some distance from its neighbours. It was only later that I learned that Nashville did not have a sewage system, so they needed space for large septic tanks. They told me that private practice created a large recruitment problem for the university hospitals. If a private surgeon wanted to employ a nurse, perfusionist or similar surgical professional he would go to the university department and offer to double that person's salary. It was extremely difficult for the university hospital to compete with such deals.

In Nashville I hired a car and drove to Birmingham, Alabama, which was four hours' drive, during which there was a spectacular southern storm. I had a good week there with John Kirklin and Al Pacifico. John Kirklin had retired as head of department, so Al was in charge. I learned a lot about hospital organization and about what John Kirklin had achieved at the University of Birmingham. Even then, although he was officially retired, he had a huge support team: a secretary for his clinical work, two secretaries typing papers and preparing slides, two doing the patients' follow-up, another looking after files, one taking care of the residents and fellows, another researching articles in the library and a part-time interpreter for foreign patients. In addition John had a biochemist and a technician working in the animal laboratory. Jean Blackstone, although a surgeon, was not involved in operations. He was an expert statistician and mathematician and took care of the database. He also employed a programmer for their computer systems. How could we compete with that?

The hospital had thirty-four operating-rooms in total, six of which were for cardiac surgery. Al Pacifico usually operated in four. Cases were scheduled in such a way that the resident opened the chest, after which Al would do the heart operation while the patient was on the bypass machine which we call the 'Open Heart'. The resident would close the chest, and Al would move to another theatre where the chest was opened and they were ready to go on bypass. His timing was close to perfection, so usually he finished his fourth case by 2 p.m. In Birmingham they had a very interesting idea of the role of surgical assistants. The three consultants did not like the hearts to be handled too much, so they undertook all the work themselves. Their residents changed often and most of the time stood by the surgeon's side watching with their hands crossed over their chests and doing very little. The daily operating schedule was very impressive. A septation was followed by two coronary re-dos in Theatre 1 and two coronary bypasses were followed by an aortic valve replacement in Theatre 2. Meanwhile a repair of an atrial septal defect preceded the repair of a tetralogy of Fallot in Theatre 3. The organization of reprints taught me a thing or two. They were kept in folders with the diagnoses in alphabetical order. Dr Kirklin would add his comments from various meetings, even filed correspondence he considered important. On looking through the folders I found to my surprise two of my letters about our technique of the Mustard operation in the 'Transposition of the Great Arteries' folder.

A young doctor told me that he was making extra money working in a nearby town around 30 kilometres from Birmingham. He explained that no black person lived there, as there was still enormous colour prejudice in the Deep South. They would not employ a black person in the hospital, as the local community would not accept it. The patients often came to the casualty half dead, but when the doctor asked them how they were doing the answer was always the same: 'Thank you, doctor. Very well. Counting my blessings.' Alcohol was prohibited on Sundays; restaurants, however, circumvented this rule. On being taken to a restaurant we had to fill in an application form to join their private club. On Sunday evenings it became a private club where there were no restrictions on drinking.

My next stop was at the Sanger Clinic in Charlotte, North Carolina. I went to see Francis Robiczek who originally came from Hungary. He was an excellent surgeon who became chairman at the clinic. He was also a professor of archaeology at Indiana University in addition to his medical activities. During the summers he would go for a month to operate on patients in Guatemala and undertake archaeological research on famous Mayan sites. He wrote about five books, including *Copan* and *Smoking Gods*, which he gave to me and which I enjoyed. His son took the photographs for the publications, which was a considerable achievement in itself. Although one is not allowed to export Mayan artefacts from Guatemala, Francis had a room in his house that was full of them.

The Sanger Clinic was organized in a very interesting way. All the surgeons were in private practice, but they worked as members of a department. They had an on-call rota both for the residents and the consultants. Operations they did not manage to do during the week were often performed as 'emergencies' at weekends. I gave a lecture about progress in paediatric cardiac surgery to local paediatricians in the ballroom of my hotel. The St Louis Symphonic Orchestra was there on tour playing Shostakovich and Haydn, and Francis and his wife Lilly took me along one evening.

From Charlotte I went north to Duke University in Durham at the invitation of David Sabiston, chairman of the department. When I arrived he was out of town and had left Gary Lofland, his chief resident, to look after me. Gary was to become senior registrar at Great Ormond Street the following year. He arranged a game of golf for me, and in the evening he took me to La Residence, an excellent French restaurant out of town. The next day after my lecture I watched them operating in theatre, and in the evening Dr Sabiston took me out for a meal. He apologized for our eating out but explained that his wife was unwell. He drove us out of town, and soon I realized that we were on the way to La Residence. On discovering that I had been there the previous night with Gary my host was furious. I assured Dr Sabiston that I was very happy to go there again, but he insisted on taking me somewhere else.

Next day I had several meetings with the department's residents. Then members of a research group presented their results for twenty minutes each and wanted my comments and opinions. This kept me on my toes, but my presentation about our results of operations for congenital heart disease without prior cardiac catheterization was well received. At that time this was quite a new approach not practised in many departments. In the evening there was a one-hour lecture for residents on the 'Transposition of the Great Arteries'. The following day I had a lunch with faculty members. When I finished, out of the blue they asked me to talk about the British NHS. No sooner had I finished my off-the-cuff remarks than I was asked about my views on the Middle East crisis. Somehow I muddled through, but it was not easy with the hysteria in the USA at the time about the Libyan situation.

The visit to Duke was very demanding but stimulating. I was not impressed by their congenital heart surgery, but their organization and

ON SABBATICAL, 1986-1987

research were outstanding. I think their research laboratories were the best I had ever seen. Everything was geared towards solving practical problems – unlike in other places where the main goal seemed simply to produce papers. My impression was that although their training programme was excellent, it was designed more to train chairmen of departments than good practising surgeons. Their training programme lasted ten years, including two years of chief residency. I had long discussions with Dr Greeley, an anaesthetist who spent several months at Great Ormond Street and in Philadelphia. According to him, the major difference between the London hospital and the Philadelphia one was the fact that in the latter they had several very senior staff people working in the intensive care unit around the clock. For my main presentation I was asked to talk about surgery for transposition of the great arteries. David Sabiston introduced me formally, but after the lecture the chief resident offered the vote of thanks. They gave me a Duke University tie and a silver-plated tray with an inscription. David Sabiston seemed very cordial, but the residents told me that as a chief he was an absolute dictator – a type of German 'Herr Geheimrat' professor.

In New York a visit to the Columbia Presbyterian Center and to attend the American Association for Thoracic Surgery meeting was on the agenda. I knew Jim Malm and Fred Bowman, the two senior surgeons, well. We used to play tennis at the meetings with Jim, Bill Rashkind, Bob Miller and Walt Gersony. They were quite high up in the hierarchy of cardiac associations and societies. As there were five of us they would suggest that Bob Miller, a less good player, would chair a moonlight session or something of that nature while the rest of us would go out and play doubles. Jim was president of the AATS that year. I was very busy preparing my talk for the following Monday. Rui Almeida, our Brazilian trainee, arrived from London with my slides. The statistics I required were not ready before I left London, so I had to rely on Kate Bull to complete the statistical analysis, make up the slides and send them to me. I think I had never before worked to such a tight schedule. My colleagues in London did fantastic work, but it was all very stressful.

For relaxation I went to the Metropolitan Museum, where there was an exhibition of Rodin and Boucher. It was very good indeed and made a perfect break from work.

Jim delivered an excellent presidential address. His son-in-law had made a seven-minute video about New York with unusual architectural shots and some crazy music to accompany it. It was excellent, but I am not sure how well it went down with the largely conservative body of senior US cardiac surgeons. After the presentation Jim invited a few people to his huge presidential suite in the Hilton Hotel, where Ronald Reagan had stayed when he was in New York. There I talked to Dr Cournand who performed the first cardiac catheterization. He remembered the names of some Czech physiologists and cardiologists such as Brod, Píša and Gans. Other attendees were Björk and Senning, Brom from Leyden, Fontan from Bordeaux and Binet from Paris. Next day Jim took me to dinner and to the theatre with his daughters and their husbands. We saw a very good production of *The Mystery of Edwin Drood*. My presentation on the 'Long-term Results of Right Ventricle to Pulmonary Artery Conduits' was well received. Lunch with the residents was one of the highlights of the meeting. Fourteen sat at each table with one senior US surgeon or one of the visiting international surgeons. They discussed various issues, and at the end the visiting professors went to the podium to be questioned by the residents. This was a very useful and novel way of organizing the event. The presidential reception was held at the Museum of Modern Art – always a wonderful place to visit.

I was planning to go to Syracuse to visit my old boss and friend Iain Aberdeen, who had emigrated to the USA in 1971. It was very sad that after my arrival in New York I received a message letting me know that he had died. He had been ill with severe diabetic neuropathy for about a year. When he recovered and started working again he suffered a massive coronary that killed him. I decided to visit his widow Virginia, as she had always been very kind to my family. After the Russian invasion in 1968, when we came to London, we had stayed in their house for six weeks.

The next stop on my sabbatical was the Cleveland Clinic. I found a schedule for my visit on arrival in my hotel room. I was to be met at 6.30 the next morning by the hospital administrator. As everybody goes to the operating-room at 8 a.m. on the dot my lecture was scheduled for 7 a.m. At 8.30 an automobile was made available to take me to the Cleveland Museum of Art. I did not know that it was such a wonderfully rich museum, and I spent half a day there very happily. Carl Gill, one of the congenital surgeons, took me for dinner at his private club on the top floor of the highest building in the city, and three others involved in congenital heart work joined us. The new clinic building had been constructed not long before, and it was so

ON SABBATICAL, 1986–1987

sumptuous that on entering it one had the impression of being in a luxury hotel or spa rather than a hospital.

In Chicago Sid Levitsky, the chief of cardiac surgery at the university hospital, arranged excellent accommodation for me at the Harvard Club opposite the Art Institute. The museum houses a tremendous collection of impressionist paintings, and I spent several afternoons there. Apart from this collection they had a superb collection of Brâncuşi's sculptures.

It seemed as though Sid wanted to show off to me, so he operated on a child, but as this was unusual for him it went wrong. He closed the wrong hole in the heart, and the patient could not be taken off bypass. He asked me to scrub up, and together we put things right. It demonstrated yet again that such procedures usually require a surgeon who specializes in paediatric work.

At the conference the cardiologists presented several very interesting cases. Their chief resident was Pedro del Nido, who later moved to Boston, where he became the staff surgeon and one of the best US congenital heart specialists. As he was a good friend of Victor Tsang he visited Great Ormond Street several times after I retired. Sid took me to the family home, a very luxurious house in Kenilworth on the shore of the lake. I was told that such a house by the lake was worth $800,000–900,000, at that time a fortune.

While talking to Sid and his wife Lynn, a professor of paediatric endocrinology, I learned a number of interesting facts. There were then twenty-eight departments undertaking paediatric cardiac surgery in Chicago, but there had been a few problems with private patients. Certain cardiologists did not refer patients swiftly, spending unnecessary time arranging tests such as electrocardiograms, echocardiograms and X-rays with advantageous financial implications for themselves. All the money the doctors generated went to the university, so Sid did not always have the funding to hire nurses and technicians and to buy equipment, as in Birmingham, Alabama. It was clear that not everyone had the same influence as John Kirklin and that in the USA medical protocols could vary greatly.

Dino Tatooles, who had worked with us at Great Ormond Street, promised to take me out the first night. He collected me from the Harvard Club, and we went to a bar. He asked if I had ever drunk a margarita upside down. When I said no he sat me at the bar with my back to the counter. I had to put my head back, open my mouth and the barman mixed the cocktail by pouring it straight down my mouth; it was quite an experience! That evening Dino introduced me to a woman in her late twenties who was the manager of a football club he had recently purchased. Some time later I learned that she was his mistress and that he had a daughter by her. A few years later, when the daughter was about eight, the girlfriend died of a ruptured berry aneurysm at the base of the brain. I felt very sorry when I heard this news.

While in Chicago I visited Bob Karp who used to work with John Kirklin in Birmingham where he was second-in-command. He was at the University of Chicago by then. In the evening I had dinner with him and his wife Sonny in their apartment. She had worked as an interior designer, so their apartment was absolutely stunning and rather different from the average American home. Bob and Sonny had twins aged twenty-three, a boy and a girl who had left home. After chatting with Bob and Sonny it struck me yet again how focused so many Americans are on making money. They do not seem to have time to enjoy their wealth; they merely watch their bank balance grow. I thought it was a very different attitude to that of many of the Europeans I knew.

On the way to the airport the taxi had a puncture. The driver left the motorway and tried to inflate the tyre, but it did not work. I had to find another cab and was lucky to make it to the airport in time for my flight to Los Angeles. On arrival I called Dr Hilel Laks's secretary who gave me the name of the hotel where everything had been arranged for me. It was very luxurious; the bathroom was enormous, and there were two colour televisions, one in the bedroom and another in the lounge. Davis Drinkwater, our former senior registrar, arranged a visit to the famous Getty Museum on the Friday. I learned that as Dr Laks was a very observant Jew he could not come to the hospital or even be on call on a Saturday, the Sabbath. If he had to operate on a Saturday as an emergency he would walk five miles to the hospital, as he was not allowed to drive on that day.

A curious thing happened to me in Los Angeles. A red light came on as I was crossing the street, so I waited patiently on the central reservation for the green light to appear. A policeman blew his whistle and rushed over to me from around the corner. He was arrogant and aggressive, asking if I spoke English and demanding of me an identity card or similar photographic proof of my identity. I found this disturbing, as one is rarely asked for one's ID in

ON SABBATICAL, 1986–1987

London. I was very annoyed and somewhat perplexed but decided it was wise to keep my mouth shut on that particular occasion.

That evening Roberta Williams, by then chief of paediatric cardiology, took me to a dinner at a splendid Thai restaurant. I knew her from my time in Boston when she had been a cardiology fellow at the same time as me. When we arrived she said, 'Reservation for two in the name of Kissinger.' I was taken aback and said I had no idea that she was married. She wasn't, she replied, but said that if she booked a restaurant in the name of Kissinger they never knew if it was him or a relative, so she always got the best table.

Visiting the University of California at Los Angeles was an interesting experience. They were using highly complex cocktails for cardioplegia and had three nurses administering three different concoctions. It seemed to work for them, but I thought the possibility of making a mistake was too great, so I decided not to introduce this practice to Great Ormond Street. Roberta was not at the joint cardiac conference when they presented their patients to me, showing the echocardiograms upside down. I was puzzled by this and enquired the reason for the inversion. I was told it was how the machine was set up and couldn't be corrected. I walked across to the machine, flicked a switch and, bingo, the echocardiogram was the right way up. I think they were more impressed with that than with any of my lectures.

After my UCLA visit I hired a car and went along the Pacific coast to San Francisco. It is a magnificent drive along the coast – around 650 kilometres – even though part of the journey was frustrating, as the traffic was very slow-moving, crawling along at about 40 kilometres per hour. The weather was sunny and pleasant, and I spent a night in Morro Bay where I had an excellent dinner. The next day I started out early at 6.30 a.m. in order to make up for the time I had lost the previous day on the freeway. I passed Big Sur, which has wonderful bays and beautiful scenery. Then I drove on to the Monterey Peninsula and its famous 17-Mile Drive. Pebble Beach has a well-known golf course, but I arrived too late to get around its eighteen holes. In addition the green fee was tremendously high. One had to hire a buggy, and I required golf clubs as well. The total would have come to around $200, which at that time was a phenomenal amount of money. So I simply looked around and took some snaps of the course. In San Francisco I met Tom Karl and his wife Angela, both of whom had spent a year at Great Ormond Street some years earlier, and they invited me to stay in their home. Angela was a nurse in the neurosurgical theatres, and Tom practised congenital heart surgery at the Kaiser Permanente.

The main reason for my visit to San Francisco was to see Paul Ebert at the University of California. I was very much looking forward to this, as his results with the baby truncuses were incredible. When I saw his department I was astounded. They did not use central venous lines to measure central venous pressure; instead, they estimated this by palpating the liver and the fontanelle. Paul was convinced that central venous lines and multiple stopcocks were the source of infection leading to septicaemia, so they tried hard to avoid using them. When they came off bypass Paul took a syringe with protamine and injected it quickly into the heart. This dropped the blood pressure to about 30 mmHg for a few minutes. He told me that this hypotension was a good way to stop the bleeding. I am not sure how my own coronaries would react to such a drop in a patient's blood pressure, but it certainly worked for them. It was incredible. Their handling of patients on the basis of clinical signs was made possible by a constant presence of senior intensivists and senior anaesthetists in the intensive care unit.

During my time there I had several useful discussions with Julien Hoffman, a cardiologist and researcher I had known for many years. All through my visit Paul was most helpful and supportive. One evening he took me to a meeting of the regional Society of Cardiac Surgery. The dinner was on the fifty-second floor of the Bank of America with fantastic views over San Francisco. Most of the surgeons were there with their second or third wives. When I met Gordon Danielson, the chief surgeon from the Mayo Clinic who was also visiting the hospital, he was quick to introduce his daughter who had accompanyied him to the dinner. He was keen to make sure I did not get the wrong idea!

I asked Paul the procedure for applying for membership of the AATS. He advised me to wait until I was proposed for an honorary membership. What I didn't know was that Paul was the president of the AATS at the time. The next year I received an invitation to deliver the Honorary Guest Lecture, the most prestigious honour one can get in cardiothoracic surgery. Once one delivers the lecture one becomes an honorary member for life. When Paul was young he had been an all-American basketball player. He then decided to retire from clinical practice and become director of the American College of Surgeons. It was an extraordinary decision for someone so relatively young.

ON SABBATICAL, 1986–1987

I rented a car one weekend and drove to Yosemite National Park. The park was fantastic, although the journey was somewhat dull, because I was travelling through flat countryside with many wind farms. In the Mariposa Grove one can view majestic sequoias, trees I had never seen before. Cars are prohibited there, so one parks up and takes a minibus. As it was late I decided to take a short walk along a well-signposted trail, which took about forty-five minutes. The route was breathtaking. The trees are remarkably straight, and some trunks are several metres in diameter.

Tom booked me into the Curry Village, a complex of tents with raised floors. They have electric lights, and there were hot showers near by. It was a great experience. I started early in the morning on a trail to the waterfalls and discovered magnificent views bend after bend. One had to walk through the spray of the waterfalls, after which everyone took their clothes off and dried them on hot stones. Although it was very cold at night the temperature during the day was close to 30 degrees centigrade. I was impressed by the pristine nature of the park; there were notices offering five cents for the return of each Coca-Cola bottle. It was important not to leave scraps of food behind, because the bears would consume them and might lose the ability to survive on natural resources. In the visitors' centre I saw an impressive exhibition of photographs by Ansel Adams, a photographer well known for his shots of Yosemite, the Grand Tetons and the Grand Canyon.

After returning to San Francisco the next day Tom Karl drove me to Stanford, where I was to visit Dr Norman Shumway's famous department. I met Vaughn Starns, their chief resident who wanted to come to Great Ormond Street the following year. Everybody had a very high opinion of him, and he seemed a nice man and a very good surgeon. Dr Shumway arranged my accommodation in the Faculty Club, a very pleasant place with excellent dining facilities. Dr Baum, a paediatric cardiologist I had known for a number of years, asked if I had visited the Rodin Museum. I said I hadn't, so he took me there. It is probably the largest collection of Rodin's works outside France, around seventy sculptures in all, so I was delighted to have a chance to see it.

That evening I played tennis with Dr Mitchell and was invited to the dinner at his house. His wife, an anaesthetist, was delightful, and the evening was very enjoyable with discussions ranging from surgery to sport and politics.

The next day I saw an operation on a child that was well below par, as the

147

department did not perform surgery on children often. On the other hand, the reoperation of an adult for aortic valve disease was absolutely first-class. I had an interesting discussion with Dr Edward Stinson, who had been the chief resident at the time of the first heart transplantation. He told me that for a successful transplant programme the chief resident was the most important person. In their programme the chief resident did practically all the transplants with the help of a staff surgeon. They still considered heart and lung transplantation as an experimental procedure, so staff surgeons performed these. I returned by train to San Francisco the next day and went once more to see Paul Ebert. In the afternoon I gave a lecture at Kaiser Permanente, Tom Karl's hospital. Then I spent an evening with Bob Szarnicki, who had been with us in London twelve years earlier. He had a third wife, Mary, with whom he had two charming children, one aged two and the other eight months old.

From San Francisco I flew to Vancouver where I was met by David Wensley, who had been with us at Great Ormond Street three years earlier. It was hard to arrange hotel accommodation, as the Expo was being held there at the time. I was somewhat shocked to discover that the cost of my room would be $190, but the next day I was told that the hospital was picking up the bill. In fact, nothing much was happening at the hospital, so I spent the day visiting the Expo, a fantastic exhibition. In the Egyptian Pavilion there were treasures from the tomb of Ramesses II. I watched the loggers' games, which involved cutting massive logs and climbing up 20-metre poles, and the Czech pavilion was well organized, with an excellent exhibition of illustrations on the history of Prague.

On Sunday David and his friend Mike Patterson, chief of cardiology, took me sailing in Vancouver Bay, a memorable experience. Phil Ashmore, chief of cardiac surgery, joined us, and they let me navigate for half an hour, which for someone who had not seen the sea nor sailed until he was in his thirties was a novel experience.

I was very impressed with the theatre video cameras that had been placed in the middle of the operating lights and which focused on the operating field. The images were transmitted on to a wall monitor where the anaesthetist could see it and also into the intensive care unit and Phil Ashmore's office. While there I met Graham Frazer, a Scotsman who had been a senior registrar in general surgery at Great Ormond Street when I was cardiothoracic senior registrar and who was by then their staff surgeon. My lecture was scheduled for 6.45 in the morning and was well received.

The flight from Vancouver to Denver went without hitch. Debbie, the wife of David Clarke, former senior registrar at Great Ormond Street, met me at the airport, as I was to stay with them. I knew the couple from when they had lived in London. The university gave Dave membership of the local golf club, worth $30,000, as a perk, so we went there for dinner. The next day David asked me to assist with a complex reoperation, and it went well. David was by then chief of the Children's Hospital – a good position with excellent pay. This combined with his income from private practice provided him with an enviable lifestyle.

Debbie drove me to the airport, and Olga arrived from London at eight that evening. She had nearly missed her connection in Chicago, and although she just made it her suitcase did not. They promised to send it to the hotel at which we were staying, which was five minutes from the airport. The suitcase arrived the next morning. Olga and I had decided to take a two-week holiday in the middle of my sabbatical. We rented a car and drove via Vail, considered one of the best ski resorts in the Rockies, to Rapid Junction. We spent a pleasant night in the Best Western Motel, and the next day we drove 40 kilometres through the Colorado National Monument, a tremendous national park. We went along the Colorado River to Moab, which is in Utah, and from there we visited Arches National Park, which has quite remarkable geological formations. We took hundreds of photographs, especially of the Delicate Arch and the Landscape Arch. It was rather cold in the evening but very hot during the day, and we ended up with sunburn on the backs of our legs and necks.

We continued along the Colorado river to Salt Lake City and to Jackson Hole, a well-known ski resort. At that time of the year it was very deserted, and we had no problem finding a hotel. Then we continued on to Jenny Lake in the Grand Tetons, which are dramatic mountains. We hired bicycles and rode around a huge and beautiful lake. We were unable to walk up the mountains as there was still too much snow in the approaching valleys, but a trip in inflatable dinghies on Snake River was an enjoyable alternative. One evening a moose came up to the bungalow, and I got some good photographs.

Our next stop was Yellowstone National Park. There was about a metre of snow in the woods around the road, and on 10 June Lewis Lake was still completely frozen. The lake is 40 by 25 kilometres. On the Lower Loop we saw a large herd of bison, also some elks, and there were always birds of prey hovering above. Old Faithful is the most famous geyser there, and I found it amusing that they had a timetable showing when it would start 'spitting' – as high as 55 or 60 metres, which is pretty impressive. Isa Lake is on the Continental Divide where water flows in two directions – to the Atlantic as well as to the Pacific Ocean. Mammoth Hot Springs were also curious in that different algae blooms gave the pools different colours according to the water temperature. The hot water brought several tons of various salts to the surface daily.

The drive from Yellowstone Park to Cody in Wyoming was very scenic. Cody is a typical Wild West town with a museum dedicated to Buffalo Bill. We concluded our trip in Billings, from where we took a plane to Minneapolis, then to Boston where our friend Peter Pick and his wife Barbara met us and drove us to their new home in Milton.

The next day Olga flew back to London, and Jennifer, Peter's youngest daughter, took me to the Children's Hospital. The atmosphere there was great, and I knew almost everybody. Its chief, Aldo Castaneda, was very friendly. I had lunch with him and Richard Jonas at the Harvard Club. I also met Ray Levey, who had spent a year in London; he was a general paediatric surgeon with a special interest in immunology, which was why he had spent a year with Sir Peter Medawar, regarded as a giant in the field of immunology. After my lecture they organized a dinner in the Meridian Hotel. Aldo invited Bernardo Nadal, a Spaniard, and his wife. Bernardo was appointed the new chief of cardiology after the retirement of Alex Nadas. It was a very controversial appointment as he was a molecular biologist and not a cardiologist. Richard and Stella Van Praagh, Richard Jonas, Ray and Rosemary Levey were also there. Next day I met Walter Gamble in whose house we had stayed for about six weeks in 1970 and with whom I used to work in the dog laboratory. I had discussions with some of the residents and interviewed the two who wished to apply for a senior registrar job at Great Ormond Street in two to three years' time.

The last stop on my sabbatical was Toronto. George Trusler had promised to meet me at the airport, but he got the flight times mixed up and arrived very late. I had an anxious time waiting for him, as I could not get hold of anyone on the telephone. Eventually he arrived, however, and he and his

ON SABBATICAL, 1986–1987

wife Connie took me to their cabin on one of the lakes north of the city for a long weekend. Our journey from the airport to their cabin took around two hours and then forty minutes by boat. It was a lovely cabin in a perfect location in the middle of nowhere. George's sister, brother and his parents had cottages on the same lake. The first evening the family arrived in their boats to celebrate George's and Connie's wedding anniversary, which was a very special occasion in a delightful location, and my hosts were marvellous.

The time I spent in Toronto turned out to be very useful. Bill Williams asked me the first day to scrub up with him for a complex operation I had witnessed in Birmingham. Neither Bill nor I had performed this operation before, but fortunately all went well. He showed me the database he and his wife Gail had developed and which they maintained single-handedly. It was very impressive. They organized an excellent follow-up programme, much better then in many European and American centres. Their database was very simple as was mine, so we were able to exchange ideas for these together and learn from one another.

After Toronto I returned to work in London. Jaroslav met me at the airport and drove me home. During the sabbatical I had given twenty-five lectures and a number of seminars and held discussions with dozens of residents.

The second part of my sabbatical took place during the spring of the following year. In mid-March I left for Val d'Isère where I ski'ed in the mornings, returning for lunch, and then worked on *Reoperations in Cardiac Surgery*. There were few problems with the chapters I wrote myself on paediatric surgery, but there were issues with the editing of those of co-authors addressing aspects of surgery on adult patients. I had approached some well-established surgeons to write chapters on their specialist subjects but found that my co-editor, Al Pacifico, was uninterested in the editorial process. So I ended up editing these chapters as well.

From Val d'Isère I travelled to Barcelona for three weeks where I stayed with my friends Marcos and Mo Murtra in their summerhouse in San Vicente, a village 30 kilometres east of the city. During this time I combined playing golf and having a few golf lessons with finishing my book. Marcos had well-organized study in the villa with all the standard medical textbooks, which made my task much easier.

One day I received a call from my colleague James Taylor, a cardiologist from London. He told me that Milan Šamánek, the head of the Kardiocentrum in Prague, had phoned and asked him to contact me about the next meeting of the European Association of Paediatric Cardiology, which was to be held in Prague. Milan, as a local chairman, had to select the Edgar Mannheimer lecturer, and he wished to propose me. I called Milan and explained that I was still under sentence to a year in a labour camp for leaving the country in 1968 without permission, and so there was no chance of my visiting Prague. Milan tried hard to persuade me. He said, 'Don't worry. I have connections and will assign two STB officers for your protection.' (The STB was the Czech equivalent of the KGB.) 'No one will touch you.' But much as I would have loved to have given the Mannheimer lecture I declined.

I then flew to Bordeaux, where I spent a week with Francis Fontan and Eugène Baudet. It was interesting how different these two surgeons were. Francis was well known internationally mainly because he had developed the Fontan operation for tricuspid atresia, while Eugène was a quiet man but an excellent surgeon. My visit to their hospital proved very useful both surgically and socially. I learned how particular Bordeaux people are about their wines. They would not drink white Burgundy, which many would consider superior to white Bordeaux. It always had to be Bordeaux. One evening in Francis's house I was introduced to his son Edouard who was studying to become a sommelier. Francis asked him to taste two bottles of red Bordeaux wrapped in brown paper so that he could not see the labels. He guessed both the vineyard and the year correctly; it was a Château Margaux from 1973. I was most impressed. Both Francis and Eugène had attended a three-year university course at the Ecole d'Oenologie and certainly knew a thing or two about wines.

I returned in time for Jaroslav's and Kate's wedding. They organized a reception in the old kitchen at Kenwood House in Highgate, which was a very special and memorable occasion. It was May, and the rhododendrons and azaleas were in full bloom. Our perfusionist Marcel Ruhier took all the pictures for us, as he used to photograph weddings in his spare time, and the images he produced were superb.

I was invited that year to an International Symposium on Cardiac Surgery in Seville and a meeting organized by the European Association for CardioThoracic Surgery in Vienna. In December I went to the meeting of the Sociedad de Cardiocirujanos in Madrid to talk about the timing of reoperations.

ON SABBATICAL, 1986–1987

During 1986 and 1987 I lectured in Marseilles, Brussels, Bordeaux and Madrid. In the summer of 1987 Great Ormond Street was running a course in paediatric cardiology, morphology and cardiac surgery in Cambridge, so I spent a week there. Staying in one of the colleges meant that we were all together, lecturers and students, and this made for a very enjoyable environment. The course lasted two weeks, and each week there was a resident cardiologist, surgeon and morphologist.

22
HONORARY MEMBERSHIP OF THE AMERICAN ASSOCIATION FOR THORACIC SURGERY, 1988

When I received an invitation to present the honorary lecture to the American Association for Thoracic Surgery (AATS) it was such a prestigious event that I wanted to be very well prepared. Originally I included quite a bit of history, as was customary at such lectures. After three months of preparation Olga asked me if I was ready to rehearse it. My slides were ready, so I felt it was a good time to invite Jaroslav and Kate to witness my rehearsal as well. Olga had always been an excellent judge and critic of my presentations, but after twenty minutes she stopped me saying, 'Over my dead body. Back to the drawing-board!' I was stunned. She wanted me to change everything. I therefore started by selecting a new title: 'Do We Really Correct Congenital Heart Defects?' I wished to demonstrate that the term 'correction' was somewhat imprecise; what mattered was the quality of life a child would have after an operation deemed technically successful. I decided to show a short clip of a football match between our patients – now in their teens – and the first eleven of Arsenal's team at the end of my lecture. I couldn't think of a better way to demonstrate their fitness.

I was to present my address at the AATS meeting in Los Angeles. They sent us two first-class tickets, and at Los Angeles airport a large limousine was waiting for us. In the vehicle was a television and two bars – the epitome of luxury. We were put in the presidential suite at the hotel; I believe it was the suite that President Ronald Reagan had stayed in when visiting Los Angeles.

Alain Carpentier, whom I met on the first day of the meeting, had given the honorary address two years earlier. He asked if my slides were glass-mounted. It was standard practice at that time, but he warned me that they used very powerful projectors at the meetings which could cause condensation between the two glass layers and as a result water circles might appear that could ruin the slides. It would then be impossible to interpret them. I discussed the problem with the projectionist who assured me that there would be no problem. He promised to bring a special oven the next day so that we could bake the slides and all would be fine. But the next day he informed me that the oven was broken. The only thing he could suggest was using a hairdryer on the slides for a few minutes before the presentation. We tried it, and it seemed to work. The problem was that I had to produce three sets of slides, as the hall was very large and they used three projection screens. In the morning I headed off for the meeting, leaving Olga at the hotel with a hairdryer. She duly delivered the slides to the projectionist a few minutes before my lecture commenced. The talk went well, the slides stood up to the heat, and after I showed the video clip of the boys playing against the first eleven of Arsenal the majority of the audience was in tears.

For some time I'd had the notion of arranging a football match between boys who had undergone surgery for congenital heart defects at Great Ormond Street and a top-level English football club. Originally the idea was that they would play at half-time, but the police rejected this suggestion on safety grounds. Bill Marshall was an infection control doctor at the hospital who worked part time as a doctor with some of the top-flight clubs, and he got Arsenal Football Club to agree to participate. On the appointed day we arrived at the Arsenal Stadium in Highbury. Clive Thomas, a well-known referee, was in attendance, while Jimmy Hill was commentator. The Arsenal players were wonderful, sometimes allowing the small boys to dribble through their legs. The captain of the boys called for replacements after about twenty minutes. Suddenly an extra eleven boys came on to the pitch. It was tremendous fun. I received letters from the boys who participated for some time after the match. One said, 'Mr Stark, thank you for including me in the squad. When we finished I scraped the mud from my boots, and I am going to keep it!' The match was filmed by the BBC, and it had been a five-minute clip from that recording that I played at the end of my lecture at the AATS.

We had been trying to raise money for the British Heart Foundation, so in order to get additional publicity we decided to feature the match on the *Jim'll Fix It* television programme. Despite the fact that I had already arranged the match presenter Jimmy Savile was insistent that, because of the format of the programme, the boys would have to contact him directly to make it seem as if he had organized the fixture. Jimmy asked me to come to the studio where Asa Hartford, a professional footballer, joined us. He had failed his medical examination because of a heart murmur, and this was pertinent. During the broadcast Savile asked me why we had boys and not girls participating in the match. I pointed out that football at that time was more of a boys' game but that we had plenty of former girl patients if he had any ideas involving them. Some six weeks later he called me to say that the Harlem Globetrotters, a world-famous basketball team, would be visiting London and wondered if something could be arranged. It wasn't long before the girls got the opportunity to play against the Harlem Globetrotters at Wembley Stadium, and everyone had a great time.

23
INTERNATIONAL MEETINGS AND CONGRESSES, 1989–1993

During the AATS meetings we often had very pleasant dinners with American and European friends. In 1989 the meeting was to be held in Boston, and the dinner was organized at the Four Seasons, an excellent hotel with a restaurant. Al Pacifico, Dino Tatooles, Francis Fontan, Lucio Parenzan, Tom Fogarty and a few others – about twelve of us – were there. The sommelier asked for our selection of wines as soon as we sat down. Tom Fogarty, a brilliant researcher and innovator (he devised the Fogarty catheter) who owned a vineyard in Napa Valley, was in charge. Without hesitation he ordered two bottles of Château Fogarty 1981. The sommelier was clearly not familiar with this wine, so Tom repeated his request. The sommelier said he had never heard of Château Fogarty. Tom asked for *The Book of World Wines*. At the entrance to the restaurant there was a conspicuous notice that said, 'If we do not have the wine that you ordered and the wine is listed in *The Book of World Wines* all wine will be free to your party.' So Tom pointed to the entry on Château Fogarty in the book to the perplexed sommelier. After that we drank the most expensive wines on the list: Chassagne Montrachet, Château Margaux and many others. I am not sure how long the restaurant kept its notice on the door!

I also lectured in Rome on homografts and on the modified Fontan operation. The meeting in Baltimore on 'Current Controversies and Techniques in Congenital Heart Surgery' was particularly interesting. I talked on 'Unifocalization – Is It Indicated?', on 'Banding and Shunting' and on 'Rastelli' and 'Re-do Fontants'. There was plenty of good discussion.

Later in 1989 I visited Deutsches Herzzentrum in Munich, which proved useful. Professor Sebening was away when I attended the indication conference. When the surgeons there presented a child for operation I questioned their decision, because we would have done something very different. '*Herr Professor hat gesagt*' ('The professor said so') was the response. There was no more argument.

The World Congress of Paediatric Cardiology in Bangkok offered a great opportunity to see Thailand. Olga and I flew via Rome and New Delhi. In Bangkok we stayed at the Mandarin Oriental Hotel, which was splendid. Prices were very reasonable, as the organizers had booked it three years before the meeting. We saw the Royal Palace and the Emerald Buddha, which is dressed twice a year in new clothes by the King of Thailand. In front of the Buddha are two deities both made from pure gold weighing 38 kilograms each. Pantpis Sakornpant, head of cardiac surgery in Bangkok, invited us to dinner at his home. His English wife, who spoke fluent Thai, worked at the British Embassy in Bangkok. We had a very cordial evening with Donald Ross, Magdi Yacoub, their wives and a few other guests. Next day we visited the floating market and the orchid farm. In the Rose Garden we saw a performance of elephants doing tricks; they had been trained to perform the most incredible feats. My lecture on 'Infant Cardiac Surgery' was well received, but because Norman Talner from Yale University went over his allocated time there was little discussion.

We visited Ayutthaya, the ancient capital of Siam, where we saw some remarkable ruins. Overall it was a lovely day, although we discovered that the status of women was very different from that of Europe. We saw a group of two or three men filling large containers with cement and women carrying them to a building site a long distance away. That evening we saw an impressive performance of Thai dancing.

At the meeting I discussed 'Palliation Versus Correction'. I am not sure if it was appropriate at that time for cardiac surgery in Thailand; it was probably a bit advanced for practitioners there, but it was well received.

In 1991 we had a very good ski meeting in Maribel, then the Rashkind Memorial Meeting in Munich. I went to the AATS meeting in Washington, lectured in Rome and in Amsterdam. I was also invited to the biannual meeting of the Asian Pacific Cardiothoracic Society in Bali, where I was to be joined by Jaroslav and Kate. The organizers on that occasion were particularly kind. My son and daughter-in-law flew in to Bali two days after me at some unearthly hour – around 3 a.m. – but the secretary of the meeting was waiting for them at the airport and brought them to the hotel.

On the third day I saw Magdi Yacoub talking to the secretary in the lobby.

INTERNATIONAL MEETINGS AND CONGRESSES, 1989-1993

Magdi was in his tracksuit, clearly going on a trip. The secretary told him that at 11 a.m. he was due to give a special guest lecture. Magdi said, 'No, I'm going on a trip around the island.' The secretary reminded him that he had promised to give his lecture three months earlier, but Magdi was adamant and left the hotel. The secretary spotted me, walked over and asked if I could attend the business meeting of the society that afternoon; I immediately agreed to do so. When I arrived I was rather taken aback. They awarded two honorary memberships of the society: one to Rene Favarolo, father of coronary artery bypass surgery, and a second one to me. I had a feeling that I was their second choice after Magdi had let them down.

The 1989 annual meeting of the European Association for Cardio-Thoracic Surgery (EACTS) was in Munich, where I presented three papers. The following year, at the EACTS meeting in Naples, I chaired a session where I talked about 'Reoperations after Surgery for Transposition of the Great Arteries'.

The European Cardiology Society meeting was held in 1991 in Amsterdam, where I chaired a session and presented a paper on Fallot's tetralogy. The reception of the meeting was held at the Van Gogh Museum, a wonderful venue. Another meeting in Amsterdam that year was the World Congress of the International Society for Cardiovascular Surgery (ISCVS). I then became very busy organizing a meeting of the EACTS in London. I also visited an old friend and former trainee, Helmuth Oelert, who was by this time professor of cardiac surgery in Mainz, on the occasion of the German Society of Paediatric Cardiology meeting.

Later on I attended the AATS meeting in Los Angeles, where I gave a lecture by invitation at UCLA on 'The Technical Aspects of Reoperations for Congenital Heart Defects'. I gave my talk at 7 a.m.; an hour later everyone went to theatres. I watched the chief resident do a reoperation for the primum atrial septum defect (ASD). He did almost everything wrong right from the start, despite attending my lecture. When he opened the sternum he damaged the right atrium, which was grossly enlarged because of a massive atrioventricular valve incompetence. He called for Hilel Laks to come and assist him. But Dr Laks was in the middle of an arterial switch operation, so it took a considerable time before he could attend. They approximated the sternum with the towel clips to stop the bleeding while waiting. When Dr Laks arrived he cannulated the femoral artery but not the vein. Then he tried to complete the opening of the sternum. They were continually transfusing via an arterial line while the child continued to bleed. They had not cannulated the femoral vein, so they could not go on bypass and cool the patient down to complete the operation without rushing it. It was an unimpressive performance.

Our Alpine skiing-cum-cardiology-cum-cardiac surgery meeting was held in Val d'Isère, so we could stay in our flat in Val. As always it was great fun; the meeting was excellent, as was the skiing. I also read papers at the European Society of Cardiology in Barcelona and showed one of my films on operative techniques, 'Closure of ASD Through the Right Thoracotomy'.

The EACTS meeting was held in Geneva, and in November I went to the meeting of the Hellenic Society in Athens to present two papers. The last meeting of the year was the Sociedad de Cardiocirujanos in Madrid, where I presented a paper and chaired a session on 'Paediatric Cardiology and Surgery'.

In 1993 I went to the Society of Thoracic Surgeons meeting in San Antonio. The skiing meeting was held once again in Val d'Isère and the AATS meeting in Chicago. From there I went to visit the Schneider Hospital in Long Island as a visiting professor. Later I participated in a meeting in Rome and at the World Congress of Paediatric Cardiology in Paris.

In June I was invited to a meeting in Prague, and I greatly enjoyed the meeting of Italian Society of Paediatric Cardiology in Naples, where I gave the Gianni Rastelli memorial lecture. I was also invited to the Asian Pacific Congress of Cardiothoracic Surgery in Kuala Lumpur, where I had a chance to play golf. One day I played with Juro Wada, a very famous cardiothoracic surgeon from Tokyo, and with his wife Christina. He was amazing. On one par-three hole he put his tee shot into a bunker, took three to get out, had one putt and then he asked if he was putting for three!

24
THE CATCHING UP TRUST AND DAR, 1989–2000

Olga and I became involved in helping doctors from Czechoslovakia experience medicine in the UK. We founded a charitable organization that we called the Catching Up Trust. Audrey, a biochemist from Great Ormond Street, was our treasurer; Irenka Trnka was another trustee; and Baroness Cox agreed to be our president. At that time it was very difficult for doctors from Czechoslovakia to get fellowships or scholarships to study abroad. Having been isolated for so many years behind the Iron Curtain meant that their knowledge of modern medical and surgical techniques was extremely limited and contacts with colleagues from Western countries almost non-existent.

We thought that we could help, but the economic situation in the UK was not great at the time and raising money was difficult. We soon learned that in order to get any large donations one first had to demonstrate that one was able to raise some money by other means. My association with the Maktoum family from Dubai was helpful in this respect.

I had operated on Mehta, the daughter of Sheikh Maktoum al Maktoum, the ruler of Dubai, some years previously. I was attending a meeting in the USA when I got a call from James Taylor, my cardiology colleague. He told me that we had a VIP patient who was the daughter of Sheik Maktoum and that I should come straight from the airport to Great Ormond Street – which I did. I was advised to address the Sheik as 'Your Royal Highness'. Saleh el Kalla, the family doctor, was a cordial Egyptian paediatrician who introduced me to Sheikh Maktoum. He informed me that the Sheikh did not speak any English so he would act as his interpreter. I set out to explain everything about Mehta's condition, but when I began discussing surgery the doctor interrupted me saying that His Royal Highness had not decided whether to have the operation done in London or in the USA. I grew impatient, as I was jetlagged and tired and thought they were playing games with me. So I told the doctor, 'Please tell the father that if he decides to have the operation in the USA I can recommend several first-class surgeons whom I personally knew well.' I walked to the door. The Sheik then spoke up in perfect English. 'Please don't be offended, doctor. We want the operation done here by you.'

Subsequent surgery went well, and I headed off to inform the Sheik. He was sitting in the waiting-room on the seventh floor, the private floor at Great Ormond Street. I told him that all was well and that he could visit his daughter with me. His answer took me by surprise. 'No, I will not come now. If I go, my bodyguard has to accompany me and my wife would attend with her bodyguard. There would be too many people there, and this might interfere with your treatment. We shall see her in a few days when she comes up to the room.' It was a very sensible decision. Later on, when I met him during a dinner he hosted for all the staff that were involved in his daughter's care, he told me that he generally used his interpreter as a buffer. Everywhere he went he felt he likely to be taken for a ride. So in order to gain time and assess the situation he used an interpreter.

The day Mehta was discharged from hospital his bodyguard distributed a handful of brown envelopes around the ward. There was £400 for flowers for the nurses, as well as fat envelopes for the anaesthetist, cardiologist James Taylor and myself. From that money Olga and I bought a stationary caravan near Malvern in the Chilterns which we used happily as a base for walking trips for many years.

I received a cheque for £50,000 for our research fund from Mehta's mother, Sheika Alia. Some years later James Taylor was summoned to Dubai. A six-day-old son of Sheikh Maktoum had a severe congenital heart disease. James diagnosed total anomalous pulmonary venous drainage (TAPVD) with a ventricular septal defect (VSD); it was a potentially lethal combination of defects. James and the boy were flown to London in a Boeing 747 with the mother, a nurse and their paediatrician, and I operated immediately. Surgery went well, but because of the VSD the boy developed repeated pulmonary hypertensive crises. At that time we did not understand these well and did not know how to treat them properly. Two days later the baby died.

The uncle came to see me. He said that the mother was too distressed to accompany him but wanted to thank me, as she was sure we had done everything possible to save her son. Then he presented me with a blank cheque. He asked me to fill in the name of our research fund and to fill in the sum: £200,000. I could hardly hold the pen. They were one of the richest families in the world but also one of the most generous.

During the following years James Taylor saw Mehta once a year, although I did not see her again. As always, they left lavish gifts with James for me. When Olga and I established the Catching Up Trust I wrote to Sheika Alia saying that it was most kind to bring me presents but as it was so many years since I had performed the operation it was really unnecessary. I mentioned our trust and suggested that if she wanted to help us with one or two fellowships that would be great. One fellowship was £3,000 for a three-month stay. A few days later a man from the United Arab Emirates Embassy brought me an envelope. Inside was a cheque for £30,000. It was a great start for our charity. At the end of the first year I wrote Sheika Alia a letter combining Christmas greetings with the account of how we had spent her money. After the holiday Audrey, our treasurer, called me. She said that the bank had once an error with our statements. There were too many noughts in the balance. It turned out that there was no mistake: Sheika Alia had transferred another £100,000 to our account.

Over a ten-year period we had more than a hundred doctors, nurses and play specialists who came to England. They came from the Czech Republic, as well as from Slovakia. Apart from congenital cardiac surgeons from Kardiocentrum in Prague, we had 'adult' cardiac surgeons from Hradec, Brno and Prague as well as various medical and surgical specialists. It was very gratifying when some of them wrote to us after returning home to say how they had implemented the new techniques they had learned in the UK. It was hard work, because around that time UK hospitals started charging visiting professionals fees of about £1,000 a month. We had to work on the basis of personal contacts, friends and so on, and people always waived their fees. We also found our visitors cheap but adequate accommodation, and the fellowship money was such that they were also able to buy medical books to take home. It was interesting to compare the attitude towards charitable work in the UK and Czechoslovakia at that time. In the UK it was normal for people to engage in charitable work but not so in Czechoslovakia. When we returned to Prague the first question people asked us was 'What's in it for you?' They could not understand that people would give their time, energy and money for free.

Another project related to the Catching Up Trust was DAR (Deti a Rodice v Nemocnici) which means in English 'Children and Parents in Hospital'. Peg Belson, who introduced unlimited visiting rights for parents to visit their children in hospital in several countries, was of great help. We did not get much support in Prague, but Dr Eva Pařízková, head of the Department of Paediatrics at the University Hospital in Hradec Králové, was a great enthusiast and a valuable asset. When we visited the hospital we were told that the parents could visit their children at any time. But in reality the doors to the department were locked and there was a notice on the doors saying, 'Parents to visit on Wednesdays and Sundays 2–4 p.m.' There was no space for a mother's bed or even a chair in the rooms. Slowly and surely we were able to change that attitude. In 1994 we organized a meeting in the Hradec region to discuss these issues. The topic of my talk was 'How I Learned to Like Having Parents of My Patients in the Hospital'. Eva felt that it made an important contribution, because paediatricians were often sympathetic to the idea of allowing parents unrestricted access to their children in hospital, but as for the surgeons it was a different matter altogether. My lecture was published in *Česká Pediatrie*, a Czech paediatric journal.

25
THE EUROPEAN ASSOCIATION FOR CARDIO-THORACIC SURGERY, 1987–2004

Francis Fontan from Bordeaux, Keyvan Moghissi from Hull, Hans Borst from Hanover and several other surgeons founded the European Association for Cardio-Thoracic Surgery (EACTS) in 1987. This was a rival association to the old-established European Society for Cardiovascular Surgery, run not particularly well mainly by French surgeons who were fairly senior in age. Presentations at the meetings often involved around 20 per cent of no-shows on the part of speakers. Just six minutes was allocated for papers with an extra two minutes for discussion. Anyone who wanted to attend a meeting of a high standard had to go to the American Association for Thoracic Surgery (AATS) or the Society of Thoracic Surgeons (STS), the two best American associations. The EACTS was based on excellence, and I became involved fairly early on. In 1991 Keyvan Moghissi was asked to organize a meeting in the UK and wished to hold it in Hull, where he worked. When the association council learned of this its members were dismayed, as there was not a large enough conference centre or an international airport in the city. The council suggested that Tom Tresure and I help Keyvan set up the meeting in London, but the members were concerned not to upset him by this. I think I succeeded quite well in this respect.

The best venues for big international meetings were usually booked three to four years ahead. It was fortunate that the Royal Lancaster Hotel on the north side of Hyde Park was undergoing renovation, and it was not booked up. Its managers hoped to have the work completed two months before the date of our meeting. Thus the first hurdle was surmounted; the next problem was raising money. The Royal Lancaster charged £20,000 a day for the use of its lecture hall and the same amount for the ballroom where an exhibition was to be held. The exhibition was, of course, a crucial factor for our sponsors. I first approached my good friend James Deegan, head of the

European section of the heart-valve company Carbomedics. He invited me to join him for a round of golf at his club at Wentworth, one of the most prestigious golf clubs in the UK where I had played with him on a few occasions. At the first tee I brought up the subject of funding. He said, 'Jarda, don't be a bore. Let's concentrate on the golf. Tell me how much you need, and I'll write you a cheque later.' We had a great game, and when I mentioned £20,000 in the clubhouse he did not blink and wrote me a cheque straight away.

Next I called the managing director of St Jude, another valve company. He invited me to a good restaurant in Marylebone High Street. When we met the first thing he said to me was 'I know what you think. You think we make immoral profits and that I am not going to give you enough money. But you're wrong on both counts.' After lunch he, too, wrote me a cheque for £20,000.

So we now had the venue and funding, and finally things were starting to take shape. Our liaising with Keyvan was working well, and everyone was happy. The presidential dinner during the meeting was held in London's Guildhall, an impressive venue, although I think Francis Fontan never forgave me for seating him under a statue of Wellington!

When Professor Ribera, a French thoracic surgeon, unexpectedly resigned as vice-president of the EACTS I was appointed to the council and soon after elected as president. It was tough at first, as I had not been vice-president beforehand, and Marko Turina, the general secretary, had just resigned, so I started with a newly elected general secretary, Torkel Åberg from Sweden. Fortunately he was an amiable and hard-working individual, and we hit it off straight away. The treasurer was my good friend Marcos Murtra from Barcelona, so the three of us formed an excellent working relationship.

Our first task, however, was a tricky one. The association had been run in the first few years from Bordeaux. Francis Fontan was the first president, and he appointed his daughter to be in charge of the secretariat. By now the association had grown considerably, and it needed a more professional secretariat. I obtained the details of how the American Association for Thoracic Surgery and the Society of Thoracic Surgeons were managed, and we asked the best European organizational companies to put in tenders. Finally we interviewed three, a Swiss company, a Dutch company and Conference Associates, a London-based firm. Torkel, Marcos and I conducted the interviews. In the end we selected Conference Associates. Diana Ambrose was the boss there and worked with several others, including Sharon Pidgeon, and later Kathy McGree joined. A few years on, when the association had grown bigger and was on a firmer footing financially, Kathy was appointed as executive secretary and paid directly by the EACTS. Its offices moved to Windsor, where the association bought premises.

My most memorable year at EACTS was 1993 when I was president. The annual meeting was to be held in Barcelona, where I had to give an address. As in 1988, when I had been preparing my lecture for the American Association for Thoracic Surgery, Olga gave her forthright opinion when I tried out my first draft on her. 'There's too much history. It's as dull as ditchwater. Back to the drawing-board!' So I started once more from scratch. Jaroslav and Kate gave their impressions, too, and I think that the final version was far superior thanks to their input.

The revised subject of my talk was 'Predicting the Unpredictable'. I was intending to show, among other things, that if the current trend of pregnancy terminations for congenital heart defects continued, and if intrauterine diagnoses improved and genetic engineering advanced within a few years, congenital heart defects might be eliminated and paediatric cardiology and cardiac surgery cease to exist altogether. I started with a picture of a microscope demonstrating Kate's work on establishing an embryo's sex at the stage of eight cells. She was proving very successful at this, so in situations where parents had severe genetic problems and a disease affected just male babies they could implant female embryos during *in vitro* fertilization. I suggested that the microscope might eventually replace the operating theatre.

I found a pertinent image by the surrealist Max Ernst of a bridge terminating halfway across a river, intended to signify the end of the road for congenital heart surgery. Michael Courtney, who had illustrated our book *Surgery for Congenital Heart Defects,* produced an illustration of surgeons queuing in front of an unemployment benefits office; Donald Ross, Magdi Yacoub, Chris Lincoln and Marc de Leval could be recognized among them. Meanwhile Jaroslav provided me with pictures of coloured fractals and complex mathematical equations intended to illustrate the diminishing numbers of babies with cardiac heart disease owing to increasing numbers of terminated pregnancies; the fractals were there just for fun.

After the talk a young Spanish surgeon told me that he got the drift of my talk but was not sure about the equations nor the fractals. I told him we should discuss it later over coffee, but luckily for me he never tracked me down.

Marcos and Mo Murtra did everything possible to make us comfortable. The Hotel Princess Sophia, where King Juan Carlos and Queen Sophia stayed when in Barcelona, was designated as the conference hotel. We were booked in to the Royal Suite on the top floor – which included three bedrooms, bathroom, sauna and a reception room – where, after my presidential address, I was to host lunch for thirty people. It was all very enjoyable.

During the meal in the Montjuïc Palace I gave a customary speech – the usual thank-you to everybody involved – but when I sat down Mo Murtra reminded me that I had not thanked Medtronic, one of the major sponsors who had actually paid for the presidential dinner. Fortunately Armand Piwnica, our vice-president, came to my rescue. He was normally a dour chap, but he rose to the occasion. He got up and somehow came up with an excellent story about a bear chasing a human in the Canadian wilderness that managed to incorporate Medtronic and enabled him to thank them for our dinner.

Early on some European cardiac surgeons established a parallel organization to the EACTS with the same acronym. Their EACTS stood for the Enology Adepts Claret Tasting Society. The professional meeting of surgeons usually lasted from Sunday to Wednesday lunchtime, but the wine society started with a tasting at 5 p.m. on the Wednesday followed by dinner – with considerably more wine. The group consisted of around fifteen surgeons; with wives and partners we were together around thirty individuals. Each couple brought along two bottles of their favourite Bordeaux. Later on the range was extended to wines from other regions; the Italians would bring Barolo, the Spaniards Rioja, Bob Replogle from the USA brought some very special wines mostly from the Napa Valley. Some of us started bringing along Chilean, Argentinian and Australian wines. The local organizing chairman would find a wine master to preside over the event. Later on we had several blind tastings. I remember one in London when I was responsible for its organization. I selected Au Jardin des Gourmets, which laid claim to being the oldest French restaurant in Soho. Joseph Berkmann, of Berkmann Wine Cellars, owned it, and I invited him to be our wine master since he was the largest importer of Beaujolais and was very knowledgeable about wine in general. After the tasting he commented on the selection himself. He started with the one wine that was slightly different from the others. He said it was something one would be happy to take to the beach, leave for couple of hours in the sun and drink with pâté and sausages. This had been brought along by Professor Vincent Dor from Monaco who had built a house in St Paul de Vence with a large wine cellar and used to boast that he kept around 2,000 bottles there. He was devastated. The wine was a Gigondas but indeed, as Mr Berkmann remarked, nothing special compared to the other wines we tasted that afternoon.

Subsequently we had some wonderful tastings in Barcelona in Marcos Murtra's summerhouse, in Vienna, Geneva, Naples, Prague and elsewhere. I was intrigued to note that often the experts – basically Fontan, Baudet, Mendler and Raplogel – disagreed wildly in their assessment of the wines brought along by members. But it was always a very pleasant social occasion. These convivial events continued until Diana and Peter Klövekorn took over the society's organization from Nicholas Mendler. Peter died of cancer, while Bob Replogle developed crippling arthritis and found it difficult to travel. So our little society was dissolved after some twenty-five years.

26
WORLDWIDE TRAVEL AND THE GLENN LECTURE, 1994–1996

I was invited to the World Congress of the International Society of Cardiovascular Surgery in Tel Aviv in Israel in February 1994. Olga, Pavel Horvath, his wife Tamara and I were there together. Dr Snir, who had been a resident with us at Great Ormond Street, looked after us. When the meeting in Tel Aviv finished we visited Jerusalem which we found a fascinating city from a historical and religious point of view. We had a revealing conversation with the Palestinian owner of an antique shop in the old town. He explained that every day he had a gruelling journey to work. His parents and grandparents used to live in Jerusalem, but he had moved and had to queue every morning at the city border, sometimes for an hour or more while his papers were checked; this he found very humiliating. Our talk gave us a very different view of the local situation from that we had received from Israeli friends.

The organizers of the congress provided us with a car and a driver to visit Galilee, Bethlehem and the Dead Sea, but the day we left Jerusalem a shooting at Hebron took place; a religious fanatic killed a number of Israelis in a synagogue. Our trip had to be curtailed; we did not make it to Jericho and Bethlehem, but we went to Galilee and later to the Dead Sea where the water was so salty that one floated without effort.

We spent four enjoyable days with Pavel and Tamara. Not long afterwards he was diagnosed with a lymphoma of a highly invasive type and needed a bone-marrow transplant. This procedure was not available in Prague, but there was an excellent department at the Royal Free Hospital in London, although the cost to foreigners was a staggering £70,000. Pavel was undoubtedly one of our best senior registrars. He had been picked as a successor to Bohouš Hučín in Prague; he attended many international conferences and wrote papers in international journals. I started raising money for his treatment by writing to all our former senior registrars and to cardiac surgeons worldwide. The response was incredible. In around eight weeks we raised the necessary funds; even the Czechoslovak Health Ministry made a contribution.

Michaela, Pavel's sister, proved an ideal donor match, so Pavel came to London and was admitted to the Royal Free. He was irradiated to kill off his own bone marrow and had to be kept in strict isolation, because when the white cell count drops the danger of infection is extremely high. He duly underwent the transplant, and all went well. Marc and I visited him at the hospital every other day. After a month he was discharged and came to stay at our home in north London. He was very relieved, and so were we.

The day before I was due to go off to a surgeons' meeting in the USA Pavel developed a fever. We took him back to the Royal Free, where he was readmitted. He was diagnosed as having rejection of the donor marrow. Michaela returned from Prague, and her brother underwent retransplantation, which involved going through the same gruelling procedure as before. Tamara and the three children flew to London and stayed at a friend's house, but her husband developed septicaemia and then renal failure. After battling for a few more weeks he died. It was an enormous loss to us all, as Pavel was an exceptional person – as well as an outstanding surgeon.

Later that year I visited Marseilles, New Orleans, Prague and the Schneider Hospital in Long Island after which attended the AATS meeting in New York. On that occasion I saw my old friend Gary Cornell in Ottawa. He had been a house surgeon at Great Ormond Street when I first arrived from Prague in 1968, and when I was heading back there that year he gave me a world atlas with the inscription 'To help you find your way back' – which I duly did. He subsequently emigrated to the USA, working for a period with Subra in Buffalo. This did not work out well, so he left for Canada and became a head of congenital heart surgery in Ottawa. It was excellent to see him and his wife Anna in their new home. They loved it there, had a great social life and felt fulfilled in their careers.

I was asked by the authorities in Ontario to advise on the rationalization of congenital heart surgery in the province. After being provided with all the relevant facts I had a meeting with the committee and wrote a long report with my recommendations for improvements, but I am not sure if they ever acted on them.

The same year I lectured at the Department of Cardiovascular Surgery in

Verona on the long-term results of homografts in conduit surgery, and in October I was invited back to Beijing to an international meeting on cardio-thoracic surgery and perfusion. In all, I had to present five papers there, which was a challenge, but they went down well. It was interesting to see all the changes in the country since my first visit in 1979. The blue-grey tunics of the Mao era had disappeared; now the young women wore colourful blouses, and in general there was more freedom of speech. On this occasion we did not visit any villages or communes, so we had no chance to see the development of the country as a whole.

The EACTS meeting this year was held in The Hague. I chaired a session and presented a video on the repair of atrioventricular septal defect using a two-patch technique. I also had a chance to visit Haarlem and spent a few hours in the Rijksmuseum in Amsterdam.

In 1995 I was invited to a meeting in Dubai. Olga and I flew over and got VIP treatment because of my earlier involvement in the treatment of Sheikh Maktoum's children. We were met off the plane by a high official from the Ministry of Health who escorted us to the immigration zone. Olga passed through immediately, but I was asked to wait. I was not sure what was going on but ended up sitting there for twenty minutes or more. The official eventually let me pass through but pointed out that I had an Israeli stamp in my passport; I recalled that I had been asked at the airport in Tel Aviv if I wanted a stamp in the passport or just on a piece of paper. I thought I had said on a piece of paper but do not remember whether I checked. So now I was in trouble. The immigration officer told me to go to the British Embassy the next day and get a new passport issued.

At any rate the ministry official told me not to worry. He promised to collect us from the hotel when we were due to leave and drive us to the airport. This he did, and at the airport he accompanied us to the head of the queue and checked us in. At emigration control he headed into an office, telling Olga and I to wait outside. We heard screaming and shouting from within, but after ten minutes he came out brandishing my passport, and we walked together to the emigration-control booths. Four were manned, but the fifth was empty. He walked us straight through this one, saying, 'The direct approach is best', escorted us to the first-class lounge, helped himself to a large chunk of cake and wished us a good flight home. Then he left. It was a memorable departure.

WORLDWIDE TRAVEL AND THE GLENN LECTURE, 1994-1996

The AATS meeting took place in Boston, so I had a chance to see my good friends there. The EACTS convention was held in Paris the following year. We stayed in La Défense and attended a very enjoyable dinner and our usual wine-tasting at Armand Piwnica's hunting club, an interesting and unusual venue.

The American Heart Association asked me to deliver the Glenn Lecture in 1995. The meeting was held in Los Angeles, so I was very pleased when Dr Glenn, one of the giants of cardiac surgery, came from New Haven to attend. As a topic I had picked 'How to Choose a Cardiac Surgeon', a topic close to my heart.

I had prepared my talk thoroughly but was wary of the reaction of the predominantly American audience. I was proud of the results being achieved by the surgeons in the Kardiocentrum in Prague. They were achieving ones comparable to those of the best congenital cardiac surgery departments in the world. In addition, in the Czech Republic there had been a rationalization of paediatric cardiac services; there was just one large centre and a second smaller one performing less complex surgery. The other two European countries that had implemented rationalization in congenital heart surgery were the UK and Sweden. So I was able to compare the results achieved in congenital heart surgery in those three countries with those of US states such as Maryland, California and Massachusetts. There was no rationalization in the USA, so, although some top departments produced excellent results, when one analysed the success rates for a whole state that might have many smaller hospitals undertaking cardiac procedures they were not comparable with those achieved in the three European countries.

At the end of my talk, to lighten the mood, I projected some art pictures, inviting the audience to select their favourite cardiac surgeon from a variety of images of famous people dating from the Renaissance to modern times. I got a standing ovation, and there was no awkward discussion afterwards. Dr Glenn came up and had some very kind words for me, which I much appreciated, and later on he wrote me a cordial letter.

After attending a meeting in Madrid, where I gave the main lecture on reoperations after surgery for congenital heart defects, the Ministry of Health from Dubai asked me to return for a few days to evaluate its paediatric cardiac services and to make recommendations. I flew out there, talked to various people working in this field and prepared my report. My recommendations were based on the fact that they did not have a large population and the number of children born with heart defects was relatively small. I therefore suggested that they pool their resources to bring together children from all the Gulf States and build a specialist department for them all. I suggested that we could, for the time being, operate on most of the children in London but that they should send surgeons, cardiologists, anaesthetists, nurses and perfusionists to us for training. After that they could start operating on children out in the Gulf under the supervision of a surgeon from London. In due course they would handle all cases out there except, perhaps, for the most complex operations which could still be done in London for the time being, with Gulf surgeons in attendance in order to learn the procedures. I was paid handsomely for the report, but my recommendations were never implemented.

I undertook a considerable amount of research around this time and published papers demonstrating how successful results were linked to the volume of patients operated on at a centre. It was hard to get this correlation accepted in the USA, because centralization of services went against the grain. None the less I found interesting data published in the American journals, in particular a report of a combined STS and AATS committee, which listed some hard facts. In 1992 a total of 451 surgeons had operated on children with congenital heart defects in North America. Of these, 50 per cent operated on fewer than twenty-five cases a year. The mortality rate was clearly linked to the number of patients operated on per annum. Just 2 per cent of surgeons operated on more than 300 cases a year; they had a more complex mix of patients, yet their mortality rates were low compared to the 50 per cent of surgeons who operated on between one and twenty-five cases annually. Another study from Boston showed that the mortality rates in hospitals operating on fewer then ten children a year was 18.5 per cent, while those operating on more than 300 children a year recorded a mortality rate of just 3 per cent. Those were undisputed facts, yet the US surgeons did not want to hear this message. Centralization of congenital heart services was anathema to them. In addition, the influence of private practice meant that no one was willing to let any cases go elsewhere, because this would reduce the income of the surgeons concerned.

We had achieved centralization of infant cardiac surgery in the UK many years earlier. Originally there were forty-one cardiac surgical departments in England and Wales. All of them operated on at least a few children. Paediatric cardiologists and cardiac surgeons joined forces and persuaded the British Department of Health to reduce the number of units to treat infants with heart defects. Originally just six were recommended, but the final number the Department agreed to retain was nine, a consequence of local political pressure. Such a reduction was great progress, and surgical results improved considerably over the next few years. Funding for the units was ring-fenced, and managers were able to appoint highly skilled cardiologists, surgeons, anaesthetists, perfusionists and nurses.

We had concentrated our efforts on surgery for infants under the age of one year, as we felt that it would be difficult to argue with adult cardiac surgeons about not operating on simple lesions such as atrial septal defects in children aged twelve to fifteen, as such patients were approaching adulthood. The Department of Health established nine so-called 'supra-regional centres' with protected funding. The results improved enormously within a few years, and similar positive results of centralization were achieved in Sweden and in the Czech Republic.

In December 1995 I was invited to a meeting in Moscow for the first time. Two residents from the world-famous Bakulev Institute met me at the airport and drove me to the city. It was snowing heavily, but they had no windscreen wipers. Every few minutes the man sitting next to the driver opened the window, splashed soda water from a bottle on to the windscreen and wiped it with a cloth. I asked what had happened to the wipers. He said that they had deliberately taken them off and put them in a safe place; if they had left them on the car they would be stolen. They delivered me to the venue where the speakers were scheduled to attend a welcome dinner, but they did not accompany me inside. They told me they had not been invited and were not sure that they would be allowed to attend the meeting because they had hospital duties. I thought it a strange way to treat junior doctors.

The meeting at the Bakulev Institute was memorable for its contrasts. Dr Leo Bokeria's office was enormous, as he was its director. There was wonderful art on the walls, and he had his own private bathroom. However, the lavatories in the rest of the hospital were so filthy that I dared not use them. The institute had somewhat bizarre divisions within the department. They had a head of surgery for infants, another head of surgery for children aged one to four years and another for children aged five to ten years.

When they took me to the intensive care unit I saw a twelve-year-old child who was grey and gasping for air. They told me that he had undergone a successful repair of pulmonary atresia with ventricular septal defect and multiple aorta-pulmonary collateral arteries (MAPCAs). I asked when were they planning to investigate him, because he was clearly distressed and not at all well. They were surprised, as they did not see any reason for reinvestigation. I suggested that perhaps he has some MAPCAs that had not been ligated and that if they tied them his condition might improve. They responded that they were aware that he had several MAPCAs but they could not ligate them because he might get a lung infarction. Clearly they did not understand the basic physiology of the condition. There was nothing I could do.

One evening Leo Bokeria took me and the other three invited speakers for a walk in Red Square. I have to admit that I got some juvenile satisfaction from spitting on Lenin's mausoleum! We were flirting amiably with three lovely young interpreters from the institute who had accompanied us. At one point Leo, standing just behind me, told the young women in Russian to be careful of the foreigners. He had forgotten that as a Czech I could understand every word. I turned round and said in Russian, 'Don't worry, Leo. I'm sure they can take care of themselves.' He turned bright red!

The following day we had a half-day free. An interpreter took me and two other visitors to the Tretyakov Gallery, a picture collection in central Moscow, and to the Kremlin. When we arrived at the ticket office of the latter the interpreter looked uncomfortable and informed us that foreigners were not allowed inside the Kremlin that day. There was nothing indicating this written in Russian at the desk, and I suspected that the institute had not give her sufficient money for our entrance fee. As we were keen to see it I was determined to get in, so I paid for our tickets and we proceeded inside. She was very embarrassed at this.

In 1996 the annual meeting of the EACTS was in Prague. I had been able to persuade its council during my previous year as president to hold the meeting in my home city. The organizing committee consisted of my old friends in Prague, who were delighted that I could help them and immediately adopted me as a member of the local organizing committee. It was hard work, but I was able to raise money from international sponsors. As far as the local arrangements were concerned, we were keen to have a successful meeting, so nothing was left to chance.

I had written to President Havel asking for permission to hold the presidential dinner in the Castle in the famous Spanish Hall that could accommodate some 500 people, and he kindly granted it. An adjacent room was designated for dancing, so that the music would not disturb those who wished to talk in the main hall. We put the catering out to tender, and Bohouš, two other surgeons and I tasted some sample menus. We eventually selected a company that produced excellent food and which seemed especially helpful and cooperative. A gift of a bottle of good Moravian white wine for each man and a rose for each woman was to be presented at each place setting.

We were pleased with the way things were shaping up. Then, about a week before the meeting, we got a call from the president's office informing us that we could not use our own caterers but would have to use the Castle's official company. When we protested – the contract had already been signed – they told us that President Chirac was arriving on a state visit and was due to have an event earlier that day in the hall. There would not be enough time to prepare the venue for our event afterwards unless their official caterers took charge, as they were experienced in doing rapid changeovers. They said bluntly that if we were not happy with this we could have our dinner on the banks of the River Vlatva! We were aghast, but there was nothing we could do. We had to concede and change the caterers. In the event they prepared a good meal, but instead of vintage white wine from Moravia they started serving the previous year's wine. I rushed to the kitchens, but again there was nothing to be done because no other wine was available. Fortunately the participants enjoyed the dinner. Most of the European and US surgeons were familiar with London, Paris and Rome, but few had visited Prague before, so everyone agreed they had had an enjoyable trip and that it had been a highly successful meeting.

27
DATABASE CONFLICTS, 1997–1998

In May 1997 I went to the world congress of Paediatric Cardiology and Cardiac Surgery in Honolulu, Hawaii. After the meeting I spent a few days in a bungalow in Ke Iki Hale on the north shore of the big island. Watching the surfers was an experience, as some days the waves were as high as 15 metres. Swimming in the bay on the south coast was a great experience, as one was surrounded by a variety of colourful fish.

The AATS meeting was held in 1998 in Washington, DC, where I presented a paper on the fate of homografts in the subpulmonary position, analysing the risk factors for the obstruction. I was also invited to Karlovy Vary in the Czech Republic to attend the European Congress on Extracorporeal Circulation Technology and to Madrid for the Sociedad de Cardiocirujanos, of which I was president. For my address in Spain I selected the subject 'Paediatric Cardiac Surgery at Great Ormond Street – Past, Present and Future'. It went down well, and, as always in that country, the social aspects of the event, including discussions with friends and late-night dinners, were highly enjoyable. In 1998 I lectured in Liverpool and Southampton and participated in a meeting to mark the retirement of Professor Hans Huysmans in Leiden.

The nomenclature of congenital heart defects varied between Europe and the USA; there was no standardization. A group of us therefore decided to put our heads together to try to resolve this. Unfortunately Martin Elliott, our junior surgical colleague, had different ideas. He was committed to Datascope, a company that had developed a database that was, in my view, far too complicated. Most European departments used a system developed by paediatric cardiologists containing several hundred diagnoses and operations. Martin, as surgical adviser to their association, had no liaison on this with his surgical colleagues.

American surgeons invited a few European surgeons to form a small working group to produce a simple list of diagnoses and operations acceptable in both Europe and the USA. In September 1998, at the First International Conference on Nomenclature of Congenital Heart Defects, held in Chicago, we reached a compromise and agreed on some 120 diagnoses and a similar number of operations. Our lists were published in 2000 in the *Annals of Thoracic Surgery*, but at the same time the European cardiologists published their long and very complex lists in the *European Journal of Paediatric Cardiology*. The cardiologists were of the opinion that it did not matter that there were two parallel nomenclatures. They said that they would map one nomenclature into the other. Professor Steven Gallivan, a colleague with whom I had cooperated closely in the past, was head of the Clinical Operational Research Unit (CORU), a research department at University College London. He had written several papers showing how mapping increases errors and was adamantly opposed to it. He was in favour of a simpler system, but the cardiologists would not shift. In the end the EACTS accepted the European cardiologists' complex lists for their surgical database, and this was adopted by most European units but not by the US departments that used the database of the Society of Thoracic Surgeons. The two largest units in the UK, Great Ormond Street and Birmingham, did not sign up. Most of the UK units used the Central Cardiac Audit Database (CCAD), so we ended up with three different data collection systems: American, European and British!

Jaroslav, Kate, Olga and myself had developed a highly usable database we called 'Simple Care'. I had used it at Great Ormond Street over two years, entering all our operated patients. All the data fitted on one page; it was easily typed up within five minutes. Retrieval of data, production of tables and checking correlations were simple. It was based on a relatively short list of diagnoses and operations similar to that used by Bill and Gail Williams in Toronto.

In 1999 Marko Turina, head of cardiothoracic surgery in Zurich, invited me to assess the programme and make suggestions for improvement. Marko was not only head of adult cardiothoracic and congenital heart surgery but vascular surgery and transplantation. He later became head of general surgery. I went to Zurich with Philip Rees, one of my cardiology colleagues. We found the situation there clearly unsatisfactory. Children were investigated and operated on at the children's hospital about three miles from the university hospital. For open-heart surgery, patients were transferred to the university hospital on the morning of the operation by ambulance or helicopter. The intensive care unit, which had as its head a senior adult anaesthetist, was also located in the university hospital. To perform post-operative echocardiogram on a paediatric patient in the adult intensive care unit was awkward, as all the paediatric cardiologists worked in the children's hospital. Good communication with the children's parents was also problematic. We interviewed a number of staff and eventually produced a document suggesting several major changes. The most important ones were the establishment of a separate chair of paediatric cardiac surgery and the upgrading of the children's hospital so that open-heart surgery and the intensive care unit could be located there. Marko Turina agreed to all this, and about a year later they had established the new chair and started work on upgrading the children's hospital.

I was asked by the dean in Zurich to be an external assessor for the appointment of professor of paediatric cardiac surgery. They had about twenty applications for the post. In my view just three needed to go on the shortlist. I placed Håken Berggren from Gothenburg as number one, François Katrien from Belgium as number two and René Prêtre, their current Oberartz, as number three. René was an amiable chap, but I was concerned that he would find the job difficult, having worked there in a less senior capacity. I thought interaction with the head of the intensive care unit would be especially awkward for him, since he would always be regarded as a junior. This was the way things were in Germany. No junior was appointed consultant in their training hospitals. I knew François and Håken well, as they had both trained at Great Ormond Street and had a very good track record of treating children after returning to their respective countries, but in the end René was appointed. When this was announced the dean called me saying that his shortlist had been the same as mine but that Marko Turina's opinion had prevailed.

28
THE BRISTOL INQUIRY 1996–1998

The Bristol Inquiry was set up in 1996 to investigate the performance of a paediatric cardiac team in Bristol during the period 1984–95. It was thought that the performance of Bristol, one of the supra-regional centres for infant cardiac surgery in England, was sub-optimal. The popular press had learned of some deaths after congenital heart operations in Bristol and published several heavily biased articles. Even the *British Medical Journal* published on its front page an image of cardboard coffins, relating this to the results of cardiac surgery in Bristol.

I became involved from the beginning of the public inquiry. It was headed by Professor Ian Kennedy, who established panels of experts in paediatric cardiology and paediatric cardiac surgery, anaesthesia, nursing and pathology. I travelled repeatedly to Bristol and prepared a number of documents at the request of the panel. I knew the two Bristol surgeons well, as they had trained for a year at Great Ormond Street. Janarden Dhasmana was a hard-working young man who had dedicated his life to the Bristol unit. He was not a high flyer but was a good, above-average surgeon. James Wisheart was the senior surgeon there and also very much involved in adult cardiac surgery. I liked him as an individual, but as a congenital heart surgeon he was not as talented as some. I felt that when he started his job as a unit director he should have stopped operating on children.

The inquiry centred on two procedures: the arterial switch operation for transposition of the great arteries and the operations for atrioventricular septal defect. Dhasmana was accused of continuing to operate on infants with transposition without taking any steps to improve his results. This was clearly not the case, as he had gone to Birmingham where Bill Brawn had excellent results with arterial switches. Dhasmana had asked Bill if he would come to Bristol and assist him with some operations. Bill did not have the time to do this but invited Janarden to come to Birmingham to watch some switch surgery there. After that he gave him his video recording of a switch operation and told him that this should ensure his competence to perform the procedure. For some reason these facts did not come up in the inquiry.

I was also unhappy with the reports prepared by the statisticians, including David Spiegelhalter, the husband of Kate Bull, one of our cardiologists. He was a leading medical statistician in the country, yet his estimation of excessive deaths was questioned by many clinicians and by other statisticians, including Professor Steve Gallivan from the Clinical Operational Research Unit at University College London and by my son Jaroslav, who was at that time the head of the Institute for Mathematico-Biological Studies there, later at Imperial College.

The inquiry panel asked me to prepare a paper pointing out our concerns about the statisticians' reports. With the help of Jaroslav, his wife Kate and Olga I did so. In my view one major problem was the use of hospital episode statistics (HES) data. The hospital-coding clerks collected these data yet did not have much knowledge of the differences between the various diagnoses and operations. When I checked the HES data for Great Ormond Street and compared them with the data I had collected into my own database, I found several major discrepancies. The HES data for one year recorded 526 open-heart operations at Great Ormond Street, while I had just 482 in my database. The HES data also missed seven deaths! In the detailed analysis of the HES data I found that four heart–lung transplantations were attributed to ear, nose and throat surgeons, while we cardiac surgeons were credited with eight eye enucleations! It was impossible in my view to draw any conclusions from this sort of data.

The statisticians also used the Register of the Society of Thoracic Surgeons of Great Britain and Ireland. Unfortunately the register did not list certain operations, so the statisticians used 'grouping', a method of putting certain operations under a single heading. They came up with the figure of thirty-five switches with three deaths in Bristol between 1984 and 1987. Yet after studying the Bristol Hospital operating books the inquiry established that no switch operation had been performed there during that period. It was interesting that the statisticians commissioned by the inquiry to evaluate the results of paediatric cardiac surgery in Bristol considered the data available to them as 'poor', 'having limitations with regard to its quality' and 'not ideal for the purpose of the inquiry', yet they persisted in using them. The HES data was used only for the years 1991 to 1995, as the data before that was described as unsuitable for analysis and was discounted. But despite these drawbacks the HES data were used and conclusions drawn.

Marc de Leval and I travelled to and from Bristol by train, often with Ian Kennedy, the chairman of the inquiry, so we had a chance to talk to him. We told him that congenital heart surgery was very much a team activity, yet we were concerned that the inquiry was concentrating purely on the work of the surgeons. As a result of this he established five panels of experts, each having a surgeon, a cardiologist, an anaesthetist or intensivist, a nurse and a pathologist. They examined a set of eighty randomly selected cases of operated infants from that period. The panels were asked to establish whether the care provided was less than optimal and did not try to establish negligence. The findings were surprising even to myself. Of thirteen children who had sixteen operations care was found to be less than optimal. The responsibility was attributed as follows: the cardiologists for making a wrong or incomplete diagnosis in thirteen children; the intensive-care doctors for making mistakes in the post-operative care of four children; anaesthetic problems in two children; and surgical mistakes in one. Although all this was published in the inquiry findings these facts were not widely reported.

Dr Stephen Bolsin, an anaesthetist and the primary whistleblower, was examined at the inquiry. The Queen's Counsel questioning him asked whether there might have been some mistakes in the data he had collected. He admitted to the possibility of a few minor errors. The QC asked for a document showing a certain number to be presented. It immediately appeared on screen showing that his errors were actually in the region of 500 per cent. He was then asked about a lecture he had given in Melbourne about the Bristol results. He said that he had not presented any details during the lecture; a document appeared on screen showing a verbatim transcript of his talk, which appeared to contradict this.

When the nurses from the Bristol unit were questioned they all praised Janarden Dhasmana, saying that when he was called to deal with an emergency he would be at the hospital within minutes, whether it was 9 p.m. or 4 a.m. This was in stark contrast to Dr Bolsin, who sometimes could not be tracked down for a whole night. At the end of the proceedings James Wisheart and Dr John Roylance, the director of the hospital, were struck off the Medical Register.

Janarden Dhasmana was allowed to continue to operate on adults but was banned from operating on children for three years. Unfortunately within a year the hospital dismissed him. He subsequently spent time in India looking after his sick father and was never able to find work again. It was a sad end for such a dedicated surgeon.

In the final synopsis of the report Professor Kennedy wrote, 'The story of the paediatric cardiac surgical service in Bristol is not an account of bad people. Nor is it an account of people who did not care, nor of people who wilfully harmed patients. We acknowledge at the outset that, in a number of ways, the service was adequate or more than adequate. The great majority of children who underwent paediatric cardiac surgery in Bristol are alive today.'

I organized a study together with five congenital heart units in the UK shortly after the Bristol Inquiry published their findings. Professor Gallivan from CORU at University College London did the statistical evaluation. The centres involved were Southampton (James Monro), Newcastle (Leslie Hamilton), Leeds (Kevin Watterson), Glasgow (James Pollock) and Great Ormond Street. These particular units were selected because they had a good electronic system for data collection. Their systems were different, however, so we were unable to pool the data into a single database. Nevertheless we could analyse the data on all 1,378 cardiac operations performed during a one-year period (between 1 April 1997 and 31 March 1998). We found that the overall mortality was 4 per cent (95 per cent CI or confidence intervals 3.0–5.2). Although the overall mortality rates between surgeons varied (1.6–6.9 per cent), not one surgeon's were higher than 95 per cent CI.

I submitted the paper to the *British Medical Journal*, which rejected it. It was none the less accepted and fast-tracked by the *Lancet*. This highly reputable medical journal had a policy that the media could approach the senior author a day before publication but they were not allowed to use any of the material until the next day when the article was published. Journalists from the BBC, ITV, *The Times*, the *Guardian* and elsewhere phoned me up. In the aftermath of the 'Bristol Affair' all of them asked just one question: 'What problems did you identify?' When I told them that there were no problems and that the results were on a par with the best congenital heart units in the world they were uninterested. Not a single mention appeared in the newspapers or on television or radio the following day.

29
THE BERGAMO SCHOOL, MEDICINE AND THE LAW

Bergamo was well known for the seminars and *ad hoc* meetings that Professor Lucio Perenzan organized. He founded the John Kirklin International School of Cardiac Surgery for young surgeons, cardiologists and anaesthetists from Europe and from less developed countries. The students would spend three months rotating through cardiac surgical departments in Bergamo, Turin, Massa and another Italian department. Then they would have a week of teaching in Bergamo and another three months in one of the other hospitals. They were allowed to observe but could not undertake investigations or surgery in the hospitals because of national regulations. The EACTS established the European School of Cardiac Surgery in Bergamo in 2001–2. Courses were held in the Villa Elios located in the lovely grounds of the Clinica Gavazzeni, a private hospital, which allowed the society to use it for its teaching courses. The committee of the EACTS developed a programme for a cardiac surgical course and another for a thoracic surgical course. Each involved a week's lecturing. The cardiac course consisted of three days of congenital and three days of adult cardiac surgery. There were three courses a year, and I was put in charge of the congenital programme. I had to select the lecturers, attend the meetings, chair a number of sessions and, most importantly, if any of the lecturers were unable to come at short notice I would take on his or her lectures. As we had just published a third edition of our book *Surgery for Congenital Heart Defects* I had the chapters with illustrations on my laptop, so it was not too arduous to prepare a lecture at short notice.

    The organization was greatly helped by Maria, Lucio Perenzan's sister-in-law and sister of Laura, Lucio's wife. She lived in Geneva and came before the meeting to help Lucio's secretary. She worked extremely hard at the villa all day sorting out problems with the students and lecturers, and in the evening she joined the group dining in the local trattorias. Any issues that the students or lecturers encountered were dealt with swiftly and expertly by her. The registration of the students and the general administration was conducted by the EACTS secretariat in Windsor, and Maria liaised with them. Lunches during the course were provided at the hospital cafeteria, and in usual Italian tradition the food was excellent, including antipasti, pasta, a main course and a dessert – a far cry from the usual hospital food offered in the UK.

The villa had four bedrooms where the lecturers were accommodated, so if one needed a short rest one could go straight upstairs. The students' accommodation was arranged through Laura – Lucio's wife, who was related to one of the previous popes – in the seminary in Città Alta, the old part of Bergamo. It was simple but adequate, and the students loved it there, because it was also cheap. This was important, as the EACTS was providing scholarships to most of the students, so we had to keep costs down. Every evening there would be a dinner for all the students and lecturers in one of the trattorias in Città Alta. This gave the students the opportunity to get to know and talk informally to established European cardiac surgeons. I used to get emails after each course from students asking questions or seeking advice about their training, future careers and so on. The participants were always very attentive and appreciative, and I enjoyed teaching at the Bergamo school very much. I was involved with it for a number of years and gave it up only in 2010 when I felt that younger colleagues should take it over.

At the time I started practising surgery in the UK I was relieved that we did not have the same litigation issues as our colleagues in the USA. My subscription to the Medical Defence Union was then about £8 a year, which compared favourably compared with some of my American friends, who handed over $100,000 a year for indemnity. It varied from state to state, being most expensive in California, and also depended on the speciality, the highest being for obstetricians, neurosurgeons and orthopaedic surgeons. Cardiac surgeons were not far behind. My malpractice insurance had risen to £12,000 a year before retirement, whereas in some US states a cardiac surgeon's insurance was $200,000.

I remember hearing of a case of litigation against Aldo Castaneda, the chief of paediatric cardiac surgery at Boston Children's Hospital. He had operated on a small baby with coarctation of the aorta. The infant had some other defects as well as a marginally small left ventricle, the main pumping chamber of the heart, and died after several operations. Aldo mentioned in a letter to the referring cardiologist that, in retrospect, they should perhaps have treated the baby as a hypoplastic left heart syndrome. It was purely a hypothetical statement, as operations for hypoplastic left heart involved three separate surgeries and the mortality rate was high; the result, at best, would be sub-optimal when compared to the standard operation for coarctation. The parents' lawyer somehow got hold of the correspondence and sued Aldo and the cardiac department of the Boston Children's Hospital for performing an inappropriate operation. The parents did not win, but the anxiety they caused a number of medical practitioners involved in the treatment of that baby was considerable. During my entire professional career I was never sued – not at Great Ormond Street nor in my private practice at the Harley Street Clinic, whereas my American colleagues had to fight between five and eight litigation cases every year.

Two years before I retired I reduced the number of my sessions and started working as an expert witness in medico-legal cases, which I found interesting and challenging work. I was preparing reports most of the time on behalf of surgeons being sued for no valid reason. The number of paediatric cardiac surgeons in the UK was relatively small – around twenty-three in total – and as most of them trained at Great Ormond Street it was likely that the opposing expert was a former trainee with us. This usually presented no problem, but on one occasion the expert for the other side withdrew and refused to prepare the report. I always felt that there should be a single expert for both sides, because an expert report should be unbiased. This suggestion was considered for some time by the authorities but was never implemented. Sometimes when reading the other experts' reports I was amazed that they differed so widely from my own, which was backed up by an extensive search of the literature. In later years the judge usually ordered the experts to meet and to try to reconcile their differences before we went into the courtroom. I remember one particular case when we disagreed on nineteen points. After we met and discussed the issues the opposing expert conceded seventeen of the points, so just two remained disputed.

On a few occasions I was asked to prepare a report for an American lawyer. The first was from West Virginia, and I was acting on behalf of a baby of eight months operated on for a ventricular septal defect, a simple hole in the heart. An operation that would take us three to four hours at Great Ormond Street had taken twelve hours. Afterwards the child bled excessively for the whole night and eventually developed tamponade and arrested. The infant survived but suffered severe brain damage. It was clear to me that the hospital did not have adequate facilities or really well-trained juniors and that the surgeon had very limited training in children's heart procedures, since he was mainly an adult heart surgeon. Once I had prepared my report I was asked to come to West Virginia to swear an affidavit. In the UK we would just send off a report in the post, but in the USA things were done differently: one had to attend in person. At the time I was recovering from a hip replacement that had been carried out two months earlier, so I informed the lawyers I could not fly out as this was contraindicated during convalescence. They told me that this presented no problem as they were prepared to visit London to interview me and take my affidavit. So two attorneys, a stenographer and the hospital representative flew to London on Concorde and stayed at the Ritz Hotel for a week. They talked to me for less than three hours. Since they won the case, which was worth about $3 million, expense was no issue.

When they asked me to take another case some two years later I agreed and asked my secretary to book me a flight on Concorde. This was the only time I got a chance to fly on that wonderful plane. When I arrived the attorney for the opposition questioned me straight away. She asked me how many medico-legal cases I did each year and how much money I made out of them. Our attorney wanted to protest that the question was irrelevant, but I decided to answer. I told the attorney I was not sure of the exact number of cases for the previous year but, as far as my earnings were concerned, I could assure her that my remuneration was a mere fraction of hers. She turned brick red with embarrassment, and no more questions on that subject came my way.

30
FAMILY AND HOME LIFE

In 1993 Olga developed a mild chest infection. I was a little concerned about her health, so I took a blood sample and sent it off to the Harley Street Clinic. The next day Dr Lesley Kay, head of the laboratory there, called me and asked if Dr Stark was a relative. I said Olga was my wife, and she told me the diagnosis was chronic leukaemia. Olga was subsequently seen by specialists at the Royal Marsden Hospital, but the consensus was that chronic leukaemia did not require treatment and that most patients eventually die of something else. She was certainly not keen to have repeated bone-marrow biopsies and generally did not want any follow-up. However, from then on she restricted her travelling because she was afraid of infection – easily picked up on plane journeys – so she travelled only occasionally with me to meetings. Otherwise she was able to lead a normal life.

Our grandson Daniel was born in February 1996 at the Hammersmith Hospital by Caesarean section. This was where Kate worked, so everything was familiar to her. Jaroslav, Olga and I visited regularly and enjoyed spending time with mother and baby. When I had my first hip replacement Daniel took his first steps while visiting me at the Princess Grace Hospital in central London. Olga and I would often look after our grandson, especially after Kate's parents became estranged from Kate and Jaroslav.

In April 2002 Olga came down with a respiratory infection. We were not unduly worried about this, but when one of us had an infection or was unable to sleep the other would usually stay overnight in the spare room. When I came to her room the next morning I found her dead in bed. By her bedside was a Ventolin inhaler and another containing the anti-inflammatory steroid Becotide. Dr Kay's opinion was that Olga must have developed severe bronchospasm during the night and that on this occasion the inhalers had not resolved her breathing difficulties.

I was devastated. We had been married for decades, and throughout the years we used to do everything together – sports, travel, work-related activities, exploring art and culture and, of course, bringing up our child. Suddenly I was all alone. At Olga's funeral Jaroslav and Kate gave beautiful eulogies – but the person who surprised everyone most was Daniel, aged only six, who gave a tremendously moving speech.

Jaroslav, Kate and Daniel felt similarly bereft. It was an especially terrible blow for Jaroslav, who had been particularly attached to his mother. This was perhaps partly the result of his being alone with her in Prague during my two years in London from 1965 to 1967. Later on, when he was developing left-wing tendencies at Cambridge University, it was Olga who talked to him, listened to his opinions and eventually prevailed in making his political views less dogmatic. At any rate, Jaroslav, Kate and Daniel were grief-stricken at her unanticipated and premature demise, although they carried on and eventually managed to overcome their loss.

I, too, tried to carry on with my daily life, despite this appalling blow. One day, about six months after Olga's death, in the car park of Highgate Golf Club I bumped into a fellow member, Sheelagh Woods. In the early years of her career, after moving from Ireland she had trained briefly at Great Ormond Street, but I did not recall encountering her at the hospital. At any rate, by the time Olga and I had met her at the club she was a consultant anaesthetist at the Middlesex and University College hospitals.

Olga and I used to wonder what a nice person like her was doing with such a horrible boyfriend. He was also a club member with a locker next to mine in the changing-room, but he never said hello and just looked straight through me. Olga and I were unimpressed by his unfriendly demeanour. Later I learned that he had treated Sheelagh well, which was why they had stayed together for some time – as this made a pleasant change from the behaviour of some previous boyfriends. However, two major complications in their relationship were that he was twenty-three years older than her as well as married.

Sheelagh and I got chatting in the car park, and she said she had not seen Olga for a while. When I told her about my wife's death she was shocked, as well as mortified at having raised what was evidently such a sensitive subject, but offered her sincere condolences. Some time later I invited Morton Pollock, his wife Anne and Tim Chapman with his wife Sue to dinner at

FAMILY AND HOME LIFE

L'Etoile, my favourite French restaurant in Charlotte Street. As Sue was unable to come I invited Sheelagh instead. The five of us had a great evening, and after the meal I gave her a lift home to her house in Islington. She invited me in and asked what I would like to drink. I suggested a brandy. To my surprise, she started frantically emptying out cupboards and rummaging around shelves in her living-room and kitchen. Eventually she tracked down a half-empty bottle of Cognac.

After that Sheelagh and I started seeing one another regularly, as we felt we were lucky to get together, having so many interests in common. By this time she had split up with her boyfriend of fifteen years, who was an orthopaedic surgeon from Exeter. Her girlfriends, on hearing about me, said to her, 'Are you a masochist? Going from spinal surgeon to cardiac surgeon!' Both were generally regarded as macho specialities.

I was not sure what Jaroslav's reaction would be when he discovered this turn of events, so I went down to Hammersmith Hospital to discuss the issue privately with Kate. She was delighted at my news; she felt I was lucky to find someone with similar interests and had no hesitation in encouraging me to pursue the relationship. In the event both Jaroslav and Daniel liked Sheelagh when they met her and approved of our association.

Sheelagh and I enjoyed playing golf, going to the theatre and travelling abroad. A year after we got together she needed a hip replacement, and I suggested that I take care of her after the operation, since her mobility would be restricted for several weeks, so, after some debate with her friends, she moved from her lovely house at the Angel Islington to my home in Anson Road, Tufnell Park. Her accommodation was spread over four floors, being a typical terraced house in that part of Islington, so Anson Road proved much easier for her during her convalescence, and of course I was on hand to assist her. After some years she decided to start renting out her house in Sudeley Street, and our residence in Anson Road became a permanent arrangement.

In 2008 Jaroslav, now aged forty-eight, developed paraesthesia (numbness, pins and needles) in the fingers of both hands. I suggested that he see a specialist, but he was not in any rush to get the problem checked out. Eventually he went to see his GP, who found very low levels of vitamin B12 in his blood. The doctor was unclear of the cause but gave him a B12 injection. As the paraesthesia persisted we arranged for him to see a neurologist. After comprehensive investigations they detected a spinal canal stenosis at the level of the C2–C5 vertebrae, and he underwent decompression at the National Hospital for Neurology and Neurosurgery at Queen Square. As an accidental finding they located a shadow in the temporo-parietal lobe of the brain. They felt that it was a benign glioma requiring regular follow-up but no intervention.

Soon after this Sheelagh and I went on holiday to Barbados, and the last day we were there Kate called us to say that Jaroslav had had a *grand mal* seizure. He was put on anticonvulsant drugs, and it was decided to perform a biopsy on the tumour. The result of this was inconclusive, revealing some inflammatory cells and benign tumour cells, but no malignant cells were detected.

A few weeks later Jaroslav developed a weakness on his right side, so the specialists at the Hospital for Neurology decided to operate. They were able to remove just 70 per cent of the tumour, as it was very close to the vital centres. From then on it was a downhill spiral. He embarked on chemotherapy and radiotherapy. I would drive him to the Royal Marsden for radiotherapy five times a week, but his health did not improve. As his weakness progressed to paraplegia – lower-body paralysis – we could no longer cope with him at home. When he fell down it was very difficult for Daniel and me to get him into bed.

He first went to the Ealing Hospital and later to a care home in Acton. The staff there were wonderful, and Kate made his room very homely with photographs of Daniel, Olga and the rest of the family. She also set up a slide show showing snaps from their holidays he could watch whenever he liked. I visited him daily, as did Kate and Daniel, who was fantastically supportive despite being just twelve at the time. During his father's stay over several months in Acton he raised his father's spirits tremendously.

Sadly the tumour progressed, and Jaroslav deteriorated; he slept more and more of the time. He died very peacefully on 6 June 2010. It was a very sad day for us all, but in a way it was a relief that he was suffering no longer. The funeral was held on 17 June, and afterwards we convened at the Café Rouge on the bank of the Thames to commemorate a life cut tragically so short.

During the memorial service for him and subsequently, when obituaries were published in *The Times* and the *Guardian*, even I learned things about his achievements of which I had not previously been aware. He had been a pioneer in applying mathematical methodology to crucial questions in biology and medicine. After he graduated with a first in mathematics from Peterhouse College, Cambridge, he obtained a distinction in the highly challenging Part III Mathematics. He was awarded a doctorate for research into chaos theory at Warwick under Professor Zeeman. After spending four years in research laboratories at GEC he returned to academia as a lecturer at University College London, where he was promoted to professor in 1999, and not long after this was a central figure at CoMPLEX – the Centre for Mathematics and Physics in the Life Sciences and Experimental Biology. In 2003 he moved to Imperial College, where he set up and became a director of the Centre for Integrative Systems Biology. This allowed mathematicians and biologists to generate mathematical models that made it possible to understand complex biological problems. He was co-editor of the journal *Dynamic Systems*. He also collaborated with me on the establishment of a database for congenital heart surgery and for evaluating the results of surgeons in that field. Indeed we published several papers together on monitoring in congenital heart surgery.

We all miss him greatly.

31
PATIENTS AND THEIR FAMILIES

Contacts with patients and their families were always a great pleasure for me. On the one hand, it was a huge responsibility to treat the children, but, on the other, the appreciation of their families offered me enormous encouragement and satisfaction. One patient I remember especially well was a four-year-old girl with transposition of the great arteries. She was diagnosed and subsequently cared for at Westminster Children's Hospital, where their surgeon did not have very good results with operating on patients with transposition. According to one of their cardiologists, most of them died. This was one reason she had not been offered an operation already, and by the time she was referred to Great Ormond Street she had developed severe pulmonary vascular disease (high pressure in her pulmonary artery), according to an investigation performed by my colleague James Taylor. When I saw her parents I explained to them that her condition was basically inoperable, but I mentioned that patients with transposition and associated ventricular septal defect could benefit from palliative Mustard surgery. In simple terms, one would perform a standard Mustard operation for transposition but would *not* close the ventricular septal defect. As the pressure in both circulations was high and approximately the same, this would act as a barrier so that the blue blood would not overspill and mix with the oxygenated red blood. I told them that their daughter did not have a hole in the heart but that in order to help her I could create one.

They were pleased to hear that something could be done and asked the risks of surgery. I told them truthfully that I did not know, as this particular procedure had never been performed before. At any rate, they put their faith in me and asked me to proceed. I duly performed the operation, and everything went fine. The little girl recovered well. Her colour changed from deep blue to a nice normal pink. James Taylor saw her a year later and guessed that the pressure in her lungs must have dropped as she seemed so well. He performed a second cardiac catheterization, but the pressure in her lung artery was as high as before and her pulmonary artery was hugely dilated to about four times the normal size. A few years later, when she was eleven, we organized a basketball match between some girls who had undergone open-heart surgery and a visiting team of Harlem Globetrotters. She was happy to participate and played well. I then did not hear from her for some years, until one day I received a Christmas card from her telling me that all was going fine for her, that she was on no medication and had recently travelled with her boyfriend for three months around Greece. I was delighted to hear her news and wrote back asking for a recent photograph of her. She sent one, and I was amazed; at thirty-six years old she looked remarkably well.

Another patient I recall was a Norwegian girl born with a defective lung. The right one did not develop normally and her bronchus – the pipe from the trachea to the lungs – was connected to her oesophagus. So her right lung had been removed a few years earlier. As a consequence of that surgery her chest organs, including the heart and the aorta, had moved into the right chest, and the aortic arch now started pressing on her trachea, causing very severe breathing difficulties. When she was referred to us I researched the literature but could not find anything to help me. I suggested to the family that I would try placing a tube graft from her aorta just above the heart to her lower aorta just above the abdomen. Once this bypass was established I would transect the aorta at the point where it was pressing on the trachea or windpipe. They agreed to this, and I performed the operation. Their daughter recovered well. The following winter they sent me a photograph of her cross-country skiing. I was delighted. About eight years later, because she had grown bigger, the tube between the two sections of her aorta had become too small, so we had to replace the tube with a wider one. The procedure went fine, and today, some twenty-five years later, she is still enjoying full health. Shortly after I had undertaken the original surgery I presented her case at a meeting of the Society of Thoracic Surgeons in the USA. Dr Hermes Grillo, an undisputed king of tracheal surgery, came up to congratulate me after my presentation as he had found it fascinating. He had encountered this problem twice before, but as a tracheal surgeon he approached the problem differently. He transected the trachea and anastomosed it in front of the aorta, but on both occasions his patients died. He was very complimentary about my solution.

In the early 1970s I operated on an eight-day-old girl with total anomalous pulmonary venous drainage. In layman's terms, this meant that the veins from her lungs did not return back to the left side of the heart but drained somewhere else – in her case to the liver. At that time the mortality rate for the correction of such a defect was around 70 per cent, and her parents were naturally very anxious. I explained that while performing surgery we would have to put the child on a heart–lung machine, cool her down to 18 degrees centigrade and then stop the circulation for up to forty-five minutes while doing the repair; I also had to inform them that there was a small possibility of her developing brain damage, even if we observed all the precautions.

In the event, the operation went well. She survived and recovered quickly. The parents were delighted but retained a niggling worry about the possibility of neurological damage. They both worked in the diplomatic service and a few months later were posted to India. Not long after their move I received a letter from them. 'Dear Dr Stark, we are happy to report that our daughter is doing well. However, we are still somewhat concerned about possible long-term brain damage. She is ten months old and only just started to walk, and she speaks just ten words. Could you tell us if she is developing normally?' I replied that I was no specialist in child development but could reassure them that I myself only started walking when I was thirteen months old and talking at fourteen months. This seemed to relieve their anxiety. About thirty years later my ex-patient phoned my office and asked if she could come to see me because she wanted to meet the man responsible for her survival. On the appointed day a beautiful and vibrant young woman walked into my office. After we had chatted for a while she opened her blouse and showed me the neat scar on her chest of which she was so proud. I asked if she was married. She said, 'No. Who wants to get married these days? But I've been living with a man I love for the past six years.' She paused and added, 'If you're in touch with my parents I'd be grateful if you could reassure them that this is normal these days. They are more likely to believe you than me!'

I also remember a furore surrounding a German boy on whom I operated. He had transposition of the great arteries, and at that time the results for the correction of that defect were not particularly good in his country. The German magazine *Der Spiegel* had collected donations to send the boy for surgery to Great Ormond Street in London. A journalist and a photographer accompanied him, and I met them before the operation, explaining the limitations of what they could and could not do, and they seemed to get my drift. At the same time I asked them to post me paper proofs of the article they were planning to publish so that I could check the facts. They assured me that this would be no problem.

The surgery went well, but not having heard from them for five weeks or so I wrote to ask how were they progressing with the feature. I received no response, but about a month later I got a letter from my mother from Prague who read German journals regularly to improve her German. She seemed very annoyed. 'What sort of son are you? There is a long article in *Der Spiegel* about you and you never told me.' I was astounded.

I replied explaining the circumstances of the feature and asked my mother to post it to me. When it arrived I was dismayed. It started by stating that in German hospitals the results of operations for children with this condition were appalling and that was the reason why the newspaper had organized the collection and brought the boy to London. That had a grain of truth, but they were scathing about their own surgeons. The feature included several photographs including ones of an operating-room and an intensive care unit.

Describing the operation, the journalists had written, 'In the operating-room there is a large team of doctors, nurses and technicians. There is absolute silence, then he comes in, Mr Stark, the surgeon – not Doctor because in England the surgeons are called Mr.' It was true that surgeons in the UK were called 'Mr' after they passed the specialist examination of the Fellowship of the Royal College of Surgeons. It was only when I received an honorary FRCS around ten years later I could legitimately style myself this way. I was concerned that if my English cardiothoracic colleagues read the article they would think I had misappropriated the title.

I phoned the Medical Defence Union and said I was thinking of suing the newspaper. The person at the end of the line asked if there was anything defamatory in the article. When I said no – on the contrary there were merely overexaggerated complimentary remarks that were mostly untrue – they suggested I let it pass. Apparently the magazine would have been only too pleased if I sued, as it would bring them additional publicity. So I just had to hope that not too many of my English colleagues read German publications, and to my relief the affair passed unnoticed.

197

Occasionally there would be a sad aspect to my dealings with parents. In the 1970s I was rather dubious about treating children with pulmonary atresia and multiple vessels (MAPCAs) supplying the lungs. I always explained to their parents that an operation might help a child to survive but that he or she would need a second palliative operation within a year or two. There would come a time, perhaps within ten years, when nothing more could be done. Sometimes I actually suggested that, if it were my child, I would be inclined to avoid surgical intervention at all. But when the parents realized that something could be done they always pleaded with me to do whatever was possible; then, some ten to twelve years later, I would receive a letter from them saying that they were sorry that they had not listened to me as their family life had been so detrimentally affected by their having to look after their very sickly child. Siblings within the family would be neglected, and often the relationship between mother and father broke down. However, I could not refuse to operate when there was even a glimmer of hope to improve a child's condition – and of course one never knew what developments in paediatric cardiac surgery might occur in the years to come.

32
RETIREMENT

I dropped two more sessions in 1997 because of Olga's leukaemia. Doctors in the UK were employed on the basis of sessions, and full-time ones did eleven within the NHS, and now I was now working seven. Olga and I had several arguments about my workload, because she felt that she had sacrificed her career for mine all my professional life, and she expected me to adjust to the new situation and have more time for us to spend together. I tried hard, but it was not easy. Even working part-time did not provide me with much of a life away from the hospital. Old patients continued to return and wanted to see me, and there was always something going on in the department to prevent me from coming home early. I started inputting all our department's data on the database developed with Jaroslav, Kate and Olga. I still attended some international meetings but less frequently than in previous years.

I finally retired from Great Ormond Street in 1999, nearly three years before Olga's death. I attended the Society of Thoracic Surgeons meeting in San Antonio and apart from hearing good lectures I enjoyed some golf with Dave Clarke and the local surgeon. I also lectured in Marseilles, Rome and New Orleans. I visited Sophia in Bulgaria for the meeting of European Paediatric Cardiologists, and I presented my database 'Simple Care' to the Deutsches Herzzentrum in Berlin. It was good to see the considerable interest in this from the cardiology *Oberärtze* (senior registrars) who were coding their surgical patients. They spent about forty minutes coding a single patient; a procedure that took about five minutes on my database. Nevertheless Herr Professor decided to retain their system.

In 2000 I attended the meeting of the Association of European Paediatric Cardiologists in Strasbourg, which gave me a chance to see Colmar and the famous Isenheim Altarpiece there. I also went to the Society of Thoracic Surgeons meeting in Fort Lauderdale where we had another session of the

International Nomenclature Committee. My good friend Jim Deegan from Carbomedics sponsored my stay. As I did not wish to abuse their hospitality I did not want to charge anything extra to my room. So when I went to the pool after the meeting I took a small bag containing my wallet. After a brief swim I returned to my lounger by the pool and the bag was gone. I spent a few hours cancelling my cards. As I did not have any telephone numbers I had to call Olga in London. In the end I had to borrow some cash to get through the rest of the meeting. My colleagues were very helpful, but it was not a pleasant experience.

Dr Martin Kostelka, my former resident, was by this time chief of paediatric cardiac surgery in the Herzzentrum in Leipzig. He invited me to be visiting professor for three days. It was excellent to see him doing so well. To demonstrate his abilities he scheduled an operation on a 2.7 kilogram baby with DORV+TGA (Taussig Bing) and an interrupted aortic arch – one of the trickiest combinations of cardiac defects to correct. He performed an arterial switch operation and repaired the interrupted arch. The baby was extubated the next morning; it was a real *tour de force*. The one problem I could see in the set-up was the fact that Martin was on his own and did not have a colleague to help, as the number of children they operated on each year would not support a second full-time paediatric cardiac surgeon. He was therefore assisted by one of the adult cardiac surgeons who had less training in congenital heart surgery. Martin had to be there all the time, and when he visited his family in Prague the cardiologists had to keep his patients alive until he returned.

I was also invited to the meeting of the Czech Society of Cardiology in Brno, and after my talk they awarded me an honorary membership; I was very touched. The European Association for Cardio-Thoracic Surgery annual meeting was held in Frankfurt where we had another database committee meeting. Most of my talks and publications from then on involved nomenclature, databases and monitoring of results.

In 2001 I presented the David Waterston Lecture at Great Ormond Street. As my subject I had chosen 'In Pursuit of Excellence', which gave me a chance to talk about my hobby topic: the relationship between the number of operations and outcomes. I had been invited to Houston by the chief of congenital heart surgery, Chuck Fraser, the son-in-law of Denton Cooley, to deliver the Frances Rather Seybold Lecture. Denton had retired, but when I was organizing my slides for the 7 a.m. presentation he was the first one in the audience. He gave me a tour of his new Texas Heart Institute with a massive statue of him in the entrance hall. While I was in Houston I was told a joke. The rivalry between Dr De Bakey and Dr Cooley was legendary. 'Dr De Bakey arrives at the forecourt of Baylor University and starts getting out of his car. A guard approaches him, saying, "You can't park here, sir." De Bakey replies, "Do you know who I am?" Without hesitation the guard responds, "Even if you were Dr Cooley I wouldn't let you park here!"'

In 2002 I spoke at the World Congress of the International Society of Cardiothoracic Surgery in Lucerne, where Ludwig Van Segesser was president. There my subject was 'Continuous Monitoring of Surgeons' Performance', attempting to persuade surgeons to use the improved techniques of data collection and evaluation. I also went to the annual meeting of the Italian Society of Cardiovascular Surgery. The EACTS annual meeting was held in Monte Carlo. There I played golf at Mount Angel, an excellent course on the top of the mountain with fantastic views. Indeed we had our EACTS golfing competition there. I lectured, too, in Rome, Vienna and Madrid. I also continued my involvement with the Bergamo school of cardiac surgery.

In 2003 I went to meetings in Zurich, Madrid, the Bergamo school, San Antonio and to the EACTS meeting in Vienna. The latter was a very successful event. I took Sheelagh with me, and we enjoyed seeing the city. We spent half a day at the Kunsthistorisches Museum – viewing the Breughel paintings among others – went to opera and enjoyed a day at the Naschmarkt. I also flew out to the second live symposium in Leipzig, renewing my contacts with Martin Kostelka and the head of the Herzzentrum, Professor Friedrich Mohr.

In 2004 Bohouš Hučín, my close friend from Prague, was celebrating his seventieth birthday, and a symposium was held in his honour in that city, which I attended. That October I was invited to the World Congress of the Society of Cardiothoracic Surgeons in Beijing; my third visit to China. Sheelagh and I travelled via Hong Kong to Guilin, but no one was at the airport to meet us when we arrived late in the evening. After having waited for forty-five minutes we took a taxi, as fortunately I could recall the name of the hotel and had sufficient local currency. I then called the travel agents in Hong Kong. They promised to talk to the local staff and arrange our two-day stay. The guide arrived in the morning at our hotel and was highly apologetic. He had apparently been waiting for us at the airport the previous night, after being told the wrong flight number and the wrong time. He turned out to be charming, well informed and enthusiastic. That evening he brought along his wife and daughter, aged ten months, to our hotel. The girl spoke and understood some English. He told us that he would teach her Chinese only when she was three. He would say, 'Point to the ceiling', and she would point upwards, then, 'Point to your nose', and she would do as instructed. She seemed to understand a great deal considering her age.

We had a lovely trip on the Li river the next day, taking in the spectacular mountains beyond the banks. They resembled the views in old Chinese paintings. The Chinese like to associate the shape of the mountains with different animals, and the guides pointed out a monkey, a bear and other creatures. We also watched cormorants fishing. The fishermen tie string around their necks so that they cannot swallow the fish. Only after a successful fishing expedition do they remove the string and allow the cormorants to eat some fish. In the evening we went to a performance of dancing accompanied by dinner. The talent of the dancers was astounding.

After Guilin we flew to Xi'an to see the Terracotta Army, which is vast and full of interest in the detail of the figures. A local farmer discovered it in 1974 when he was digging his field, and he was sitting at the entrance when we arrived; for $10 one could have one's picture taken with him. When Sheelagh wanted her photograph taken after mine he asked for a second $10! He was a good businessman. Terracotta Warriors and Horses is a collection of terracotta sculptures depicting the armies of Qin Shi Huang, the first Emperor of China. It is a form of funerary art buried with the emperor in 210–209 BC whose purpose was to protect the emperor in his afterlife. It is estimated that in the three pits containing the Terracotta Army there were more than 8,000 soldiers, 130 chariots with 520 horses and 150 cavalry, the majority of which are still buried.

In Xi'an we had a helpful female guide who was very well informed and spoke excellent English, like many we encountered; tourism was a popular career choice. From there we flew to Beijing to attend the meeting. There were only three foreign guests there: Denton Cooley from Houston, Stuart Jamieson, a transplant surgeon originally from Zimbabwe who had trained in London but was by this time working in San Diego, and myself. We were each given a penthouse suite with a large television screen in a mid-range hotel in Beijing. The reason for this was that they wanted to make the hotel affordable for the Chinese doctors in attendance. The breakfasts were Chinese-style and none too appetizing, but overall the accommodation was adequate.

On the days I was not presenting papers we were taken to see the sights. Dr Wei-guo Ma, our interpreter and guide, was very keen to train at Great Ormond Street and did absolutely everything for us. He was driving his wife's large American automobile. She worked for an insurance company, so she could afford it, while for doctors ownership of such a car was out of reach. We went to the Forbidden City with the Cooleys. Denton was great with the locals, patient and understanding. His wife Louisa, on the other hand, who was eighty, was a typical American wife. Seeing one of the temples she said, tongue in cheek, 'I think I will ask my next husband to build me a house like this.' At one point our guide wanted to show us something a short distance away; as the Cooleys were rather slow, he asked them to wait for us, saying that we would be back in ten minutes. We were late by a few minutes, and Louisa was furious. 'We do not wait for people,' she told the guide frostily. The night of the main banquet the ballroom doors did not open on time. Louisa commented, 'They'd better get their act together before the Olympics. You can't even get a cocktail here!'

During the dinner I found myself sitting next to Stuart Jamieson's wife. Sheelagh muttered quietly to me that she had evidently undergone extensive plastic surgery: nose, lips, facelift and the rest. Having anaesthetized for cosmetic surgeons she had a good eye for spotting such procedures. One of the first subjects Dr Jamieson's wife discussed with me was Christmas presents. I asked her what she would give her husband as a present. He wanted something very badly, she said. When I asked what, she said a helicopter. She mentioned their previous year's trip to Istanbul. I asked if they had bought any carpets there. Because they had a large ranch with eighty rooms an hour's flight from San Diego they had decided to buy a carpet for every single room. I thought that was impressive American ostentation.

In January 2005 Jeff Jacobs invited me as a visiting professor to St Petersburg, where we met his colleague Dr Quintenezza who was not only a good surgeon but an excellent golfer. At the end of our trip Jeff arranged for us a two-day stay in a good hotel on the beach, courtesy of the Department of Cardiac Surgery. Around that time Sheelagh and I attended the Society of Thoracic Surgeons meeting in Tampa, Florida. We visited Salvador Dalí's museum, which houses the largest collection of the artist's pictures outside Spain. Sheelagh left her camera in the toilet at the museum and discovered her loss only when we returned to the hotel. We went back, but by then it had been found and locked in the safe of the director's office – and he had gone home for the day. Next day we asked a taxi driver if he would kindly pick it up for us, and he did. He was a very pleasant man known locally as Three Stools Tony, as he had previously been so overweight that he needed three stools while sitting at the bar. He had bought an exercise machine and gone on a strict diet. We could not recognize him from the photograph he showed us from his fat phase.

The purchase of our holiday flat in Mandelieu near Cannes in southern France came about when we saw that French property companies were exhibiting at the Holiday Inn in Hammersmith in April 2005. We had no intention of buying anything, but out of curiosity we went. The company in question had many ways to entice the customers. They offered to fly us to Nice, arrange a hotel and show us what was available with no strings attached. We thought that two days in the Côte d'Azur would be agreeable enough, so we accepted. We originally were considering old traditional hilltop Provençal houses. We saw a few, but in the evening, back at the hotel, I had second thoughts. I thought, what would happen if the roof started to leak? It was bad enough if it happened in London, but a thousand miles away was another matter entirely. So in the morning we asked the sales rep, Shirley, to show us some modern flats. She was a very likeable Northern Irish woman who drove us around on behalf of the estate agents, and we were to become friends. She showed us a new development of apartments in a medium-size development above Mandelieu, about six kilometres west of Cannes. The building had not yet been constructed, but we bought it off plan which gave us about 25 per cent discount, and we were able to change a few things in the architectural designs, select our own tiles and so on. The building was completed in eighteen months, as originally promised.

One day in May 2005 I opened a good bottle of wine, put on some nice music, cooked a special dinner for us and presented Sheelagh with a diamond engagement ring from Tiffany's. She was delighted but within a few minutes asked if I didn't agree that the diamond was a bit small for her chunky fingers. So it was decided that she would go along to Tiffany's and exchange it. The staff there were unhelpful, despite the fact that she made two trips. Indeed they were very high-handed in their attitude and became irritated with her. Eventually they told her that they had a policy of taking back goods within twenty-eight days of purchase. This came as a surprise, because she had been unaware that it could be returned. She phoned me nervously to ask when I had bought the ring. I told her twenty-five days earlier, and she was highly relieved. She left the ring at the store, and the staff said they would have to have it examined by a gemologist to make sure it was undamaged.

A few days later we left London for a week in Istanbul, which proved a fantastic holiday. Our new friend Shirley had given us a recommendation for a good restaurant where we went to eat, although our taxi driver that evening was a maniac. I think that I was never so scared during any journey.

We visited a gold souk, where we saw a number of rings and diamonds. I was particularly interested in one in a shop run by a Christian. I chatted to him and tried to persuade Sheelagh to buy it, but she wanted to see more before deciding.

In front of the Blue Mosque an affable young man offered to show us around. He spoke excellent English, so we agreed. After the visit to the mosque he suggested that we go to his uncle's carpet shop. There we purchased a lovely rug, and he asked if we were looking for anything else to take home. Sheelagh told him that we hadn't been thinking of buying a carpet but were looking for an engagement ring. Our friend immediately suggested a visit to his brother's jewellery shop. There we found a beautiful diamond which they promised to set in a ring the next day, but they did not manage to do this, so we bought the stone to take back home. On the plane to London Sheelagh started panicking. 'What if it's glass and not a diamond at all?' she exclaimed.

In London she took the gem to a reputable jeweller, who confirmed that it was definitely a true diamond, perhaps not as good quality as the seller had made out, but, still, she was very happy with it and had the jeweller set it into a handsome ring.

This was not the end of the saga, however. Some months later she was doing a list of epidural anaesthesia that entailed scrubbing up, so she put the ring in the pocket of her scrub suit. Afterwards she changed quickly and went out with her team for a drink. It was only later that evening she realized she had forgotten to recover her jewellery. She called the hospital but was told that the scrub suits had already been sent to the laundry in Brixton. 'The ring's down the plughole, love,' they told her.

One of her registrars had bought a beautiful diamond ring in Dubai that cost half the price of one in the West. Because her cousin lived in Dubai at that time Sheelagh found a cheap air ticket and flew straight out. She came back three days later with a ring set with a diamond twice the size of the one I had originally bought her. Through a friend in Ireland she managed to get a receipt for the original ring for insurance purposes, which covered the cost of the new and beautiful ring. So we were engaged, and the ring has been in her possession ever since!

In June 2005 we had two weeks' holiday on a golf course at Sperone in Corsica. The course was beautiful with lovely views, some holes overlooking the aquamarine sea and some facing inland. We played and practised a great deal, so Sheelagh managed to win several competitions in Highgate after our return. In July I took Daniel on holiday in Dorset, where I rented a cottage, and my friends from Prague, Franta and Zdena Piťha, joined us for a week, and Jaroslav and Kate came down for the weekend. We had a wonderful time with lots of good walks and swims and generally enjoyed ourselves. That year I started playing golf for the Highgate seniors, which was very enjoyable. We had matches with several north London clubs, Harrow School, Finchley, Stanmore, North Middlesex and others. Usually we had a home match and then a return match at their club.

Meanwhile I continued organizing the courses and lecturing at the Bergamo school. In October 2005 we went on a long trip to Australia. We travelled via Singapore, where we spent three days with Seong Saw, a former Great Ormond Street resident, who looked after us. We had several memorable meals, especially ones involving seafood, and we went to a traditional Japanese restaurant, where they cook the meals on a hotplate in front of you. I gave two lectures in the hospital there and did the teaching ward round. Then we flew to Sydney, where our travel agent in Bath arranged for us to stay in a lovely apartment overlooking the Opera House and Harbour Bridge. I had found what sounded like a good hotel on the internet, but when I checked with Tim Giles, our travel agent, he told me that although it was OK he would recommend more highly another about 200 metres further on, which was not only cheaper but had an apartment with a kitchenette, bedroom and large sitting-room. He certainly knew his stuff.

One night we went to the opera to see *Romeo and Juliet*, which was an unforgettable experience. The Opera House is beautiful from the outside, but the interior is equally stunning.

From Sydney we flew to Brisbane, where we stayed with Homayoun Jalali, another former Great Ormond Street resident, by then chief of paediatric cardiac surgery in Brisbane. He took us for a two-day meeting of the Australian Cardiothoracic Society in Noosa Beach, reputedly the finest beach in Australia. We enjoyed both the meeting and the lovely beach, which stretched for kilometres. From there we flew to Cairns and on to Lizard Island, which was heavenly. There was just one hotel on the island, which consisted of a series of bungalows located on the beach. On arrival we had a bottle of champagne in our room, as Tim Giles had arranged our holiday as a honeymoon when he heard about our engagement. The bungalow was 10 metres from the water's edge, and we could borrow a boat with an outboard motor and go around the island. We snorkelled, swam and had a wonderful time. Back in Cairns we met Oliver, Sheelagh's brother, and his wife Cecilia and went with them north to the jungle in Daintree.

After a few very pleasant days including golf we flew to Melbourne, which we preferred to Sydney. There seemed to be much more culture, and we considered it a very interesting city. Then we flew to Fiji, where we stayed once more in a deluxe bungalow – but there was no champagne in the room on arrival. I called the manager and asked what had gone wrong. He apologized and was very swift in sending a bottle to our room. He told us we had also been upgraded. Our bungalow was the same as that where Prince Charles stayed when he visited Fiji – but he was there for just a few hours to have an egg-and-cress sandwich and to change his shirt. Sheelagh then started pulling the manager's leg, as she thought he seemed the gullible sort. She said that now that we were married we were hoping for a child. He told us that Abraham had a child with Sarah when they were in their eighties. It all depended on faith, he assured us.

In Fiji we met Epele Nailatikau, who used to be a member of Highgate Golf Club. He was Fiji's high commissioner in London and then became speaker of the Fiji parliament, thus a very important man; he later went on to become president. He invited us to his club to play golf and have dinner with him. In return we invited him to our hotel for a meal. When I booked the table I suggested 8.30 p.m., but they told me the kitchen closed at 8.

I mentioned that we were having a very important guest, a Mr Nailatikau. Their attitude changed immediately. They would keep the kitchen open as long as necessary, they told us. We had a delightful dinner and some interesting discussions. The last day we took a taxi to the airport. When we got out two huge Fijians asked me if I was Dr Stark. They took our suitcases and checked us in and took us to the lounge. Epele had sent them. When we returned to England someone at the golf club told us an entertaining story about him. He used to play on Saturdays and liked to have a drink or two at the bar afterwards. So he was usually late coming home. When his wife wondered why he told her the club was far away. But one Sunday they went there for lunch. Epele's chauffeur had to drive around in circles to convince her that the club really was a long way away!

From Fiji we flew via San Francisco to Portland, Oregon, where we stayed with Sheelagh's sister Bronagh. Even though we were only there for a day or two we managed to meet her family, play some golf and to go for a drive along the Willamette river, enjoying the astounding Oregon scenery before we flew to London to complete our round-the-world trip.

In April 2006 I attended the American Association for Thoracic Surgery meeting in Philadelphia. While there I visited the Barnes Collection and the Longwood Gardens near Philadelphia. The Barnes Collection is a very impressive collection of paintings by French impressionists amassed by a businessman who made his money from drugs to treat syphilis. Unfortunately the pictures were exhibited very close together on the walls, sometimes in three or four rows, one above the other. It did not make a very good aesthetic impression. Nevertheless the collection was amazing. One generally saw just one floor at a time, since one required a second ticket to visit another floor. It was only recently that the family had to make it more freely accessible under threat of paying more taxes. My good friend Jeff Dunn booked my tickets well in advance, so I had no problem in this respect.

My sister and her two granddaughters came to visit us in July. I booked a cottage in Norfolk, and we went there with Daniel for two weeks. It was delightful, as it gave them a taste of the English countryside and seaside, and for my grandson it was a welcome break. We made several interesting trips, including one to the local zoo. I continued my involvement with the Bergamo school and attended the European Association of Cardio-Thoracic Surgery meeting in Stockholm.

In October that year Sheelagh and I had a superb holiday in Peru, Ecuador and the Galapagos Islands. We flew to Lima via Madrid and then on to Cusco, which is very high, about 3,300 metres, and despite the fact that we were taking Diamox I developed mild mountain sickness. When we went to a restaurant one evening I became dizzy and felt a bit sick, but fortunately I had recovered by the following day. We learned later that the two most exquisite hotels had piped oxygen in some rooms for this reason. We did some shopping, buying some beautiful Peruvian sweaters for the two of us and also for Jaroslav and for Sheelagh's brother Oliver. Our visit to Machu Picchu was amazing. It is a fifteenth-century Incan site located at an altitude of 2,400 metres and was discovered only in 1911 by an American historian, Hiram Bingham. The Incas were masters of the construction technique called ashlar, in which blocks of stone are cut to fit together tightly without mortar. The site consisted of about two hundred buildings, and how they managed to get all the materials from the valley up the mountain remains a mystery.

From Machu Picchu we visited the sacred valley called Urubamba and the Incan archaeological site at Moray with its striking terraces and the town of Písac. It was market day, so we managed to buy some eye-catching tapestries which we later put on the walls of our flat in Mandelieu. We then flew to Lima and visited the museum of erotic art where I took a series of photographs that amused our friends in London. From Lima we moved to Quito, formally San Francisco de Quito, which is the capital city of Ecuador and at 2,800 metres is the highest capital city in the world. The Cathedral of Quito and the church of San Francisco on the Plaza de San Francisco were the two most interesting religious sites that we visited.

We reached the Equator and stayed in a hacienda in the highlands and then visited the Cuicocha Lake. The best part of the holiday was probably the seven days on a boat sailing around the Galapagos Islands. Seeing the animals there was an incredible experience. Humans do not frighten them, so one can get very close. The Charles Darwin Research Station is located on one of the islands. They had a huge number of young tortoises threatened with extinction because eggs were damaged or eaten by rats and donkeys. So the researchers collected the eggs, incubated them and after about four years they put the young tortoises back on their original islands. They also had Lonesome George, a very old male tortoise they guessed was about 150 years old. They would have liked him to mate him, but he was not interested – despite the tortoise pornography a Swiss researcher showed him!

During that year we took a bridge course at the Acol Bridge School and started playing regularly with our friends the Chaumetons. We also continued to have private lessons with the Chaumetons every three weeks so as to keep our bad habits at bay. Despite starting so late in life we enjoyed playing the game a great deal.

My friends from Prague invited me in January 2007 to a meeting of paediatric cardiologists in Poděbrady Spa. It was not far from Prague, and the meeting was very enjoyable. Afterwards Milan Šamánek presented a paper on the beneficial effects of wine on the heart.

The following April I was playing in a golf competition when I felt a strange pressure in my chest. I was two up with three to play, so I thought we could go on. But soon it became clear that I could not continue. I realized that I was having a coronary, so I went back to the clubhouse and asked for an aspirin and a double whisky. As I was sure I was having a heart attack I called my successor at Great Ormond Street, Victor Tsang, asking him where I should go. He was astounded, saying, 'Jarda, you are not the type for a coronary!' Anyway he suggested going to the emergency room at University College Hospital, which he thought would be the best place to sort me out; he guessed they would probably transfer me to the Heart Hospital. He phoned them to say that I would be arriving shortly. Michael Sandler, my golfing opponent, was somewhat reluctant to drive me to the hospital, as he was apprensive about the consequences of a non-medical person being in charge of escorting me there. However, I did not wish to wait for an ambulance, which might mean waiting for half an hour and being driven to the nearest hospital – which I really did not want. Eventually I persuaded him to take me to UCH.

I called Sheelagh from his car, but her phone went straight to answering machine. I finally managed to get hold of her just before we arrived. I asked why her phone had been switched off, and she replied, 'I'm out drinking with some girlfriends. What's the fuss?' When I told her I was on my way to UCH with a coronary she was staggered. On arriving at A&E I found a long admission queue. I went straight to the window. I was told to go to the end of the queue, but when I explained that they were expecting me the clerk called for a wheelchair and they took me straight to a cubicle. A kind nurse tried to put up a drip, but as my veins had shut down she found it hard to insert the needle.

At this point Sheelagh stormed in, saw the nurse having trouble and said, 'Give it to me. I do this all the time.' Her intervention did the trick, and the drip was up. Working as an anaesthetist until her retirement she knew exactly what to do. They were giving me very small increments of morphine, which had little or no effect on the pain, so Sheelagh took the syringe and gave me a more substantial dose, but even that did not relieve the pain. Shortly afterwards the ambulance took me to the Heart Hospital, and I was taken straight to the catheterization laboratory. Dr David Brull, the cardiologist there, said, 'A little scratch coming up', and in no time I saw on the screen that the tip of the catheter was in my left main coronary artery. They found two stenoses, dilated them and inserted two stents – all within ninety minutes of me making the diagnosis. It was not until I had the dilation and stenting of my coronaries that the pain was relieved. The heart did not have a chance to suffer any ill effects, which was excellent, and I recovered well. My friends at the golf club asked me subsequently to give them the telephone numbers I had used on that occasion in case something similar happened to them.

We spent two weeks in May 2007 and another two weeks in September in Mandelieu. In June and October I went again to Bergamo. From there we visited Venice, which was most enjoyable. We visited the museums, galleries and churches and had some excellent meals. We went to Torcello and Murano and, all in all, enjoyed Venice very much. In July I took Daniel for ten days to Prague and Senohraby, which he really appreciated. He was keen to explore his Czech origins probably because he was more mature by now. In September the European Association of Cardio-Thoracic Surgery meeting was held in Geneva. We visited my Czech friends Eva and Ivan Lehraus and went to Anzère in the mountains to see the Deenys, relatives of Sheelagh. As my back had been bothering me my friend Honza Lehovsky did a L2–L4 decompression on me in Stanmore Hospital in the November of that year.

33
HOUSE RENOVATION AND FURTHER HOLIDAYS 2008–2015

In 2008 we decided to make some major improvements to our house in Tufnell Park. Our friend Duncan Cardow was an architect, and he provided the plans for the alterations, then a group of Polish builders under Rafal did the work. They were superb, keeping to the time schedule and to their financial estimate. The alterations consisted of an extension to the dining-room and knocking down a wall between the kitchen and the dining area, making it open plan. Duncan also suggested getting rid of the larder and an outside toilet so that we could have a good view of the garden from the kitchen. The space thus gained was used to build a utility room and a downstairs shower and toilet. Duncan said to Sheelagh, 'Let's face it. In a year Jarda won't be able to make it to the first floor.' I thought I would kill him when I heard this.

In the front room we built shelves for a large library. We placed our art books and catalogues from exhibitions there. The entire house was rewired, and some changes were made upstairs. Fortunately we were able to move to Sheelagh's house in Sudeley Street, Islington, to escape all the noise and dust; there we stayed for six months. Sheelagh and our Filipina cleaner Lita packed all our effects into boxes in Anson Road, and Rafal moved them from room to room as required.

The result was wonderful, as the house was transformed into a more modern one. A skylight was installed in the extension, and everything became light and bright. We asked Moira Latham, a garden designer, to redesign the garden. The lawn, because of its north-facing position, was never great, so we paved it and placed a garden table with six chairs there. Moira's design proved excellent, and something is usually flowering somewhere in the garden all the year round.

In February 2008 we went to Mandelieu to see the mimosas in bloom.

HOUSE RENOVATIONS AND FURTHER HOLIDAYS, 2008–2015

It was an extraordinary sight, as the hills around Cannes were covered with beautiful yellow flowering trees with a wonderful scent. The drive from Mandelieu to the golf course in Grasse was like a journey through a yellow tunnel. In fact Mandelieu is known as the Capital of Mimosas. In May and September we returned there, the Bergamo course being held in June and September.

In July Jaroslav, Daniel and I went to the Czech Republic, to Prague and Senohraby but also to Hradec Králové and Pardubice, where Jaroslav had been born. We also visited Rychnov nad Kněžnou, where I used to work and where Jaroslav spent the first three years of his life. It was a delightful visit, and we went for a long walk with our friend Radko Vaněk in the Orlické Mountains and enjoyed seeing familiar old sights.

In August Sheelagh and I visited Carlo and Imgaard Kallfelz in Hanover. We went to celebrate their wedding anniversary and played some golf. They were old friends who had been tremendously helpful at the time of leaving Czechoslovakia after the Russian invasion, and our visit was highly enjoyable. The European Association of Cardio-Thoracic Surgeons meeting that year was held in Lisbon, where we had a reunion of former Great Ormond Street residents and we played some golf with Dave Clarke and the Lisbon chief of cardiac surgery.

In November John and Carol Newman invited us to Barbados. We spent a week in Little Good Harbour and then a week with them. Golfing at Westmoreland was superb, and we had a lovely time. In March 2009 I had a re-replacement of my right hip, which was a major operation. My femur was bent, so in order to get the old prosthesis out the surgeon, Sarah Muirhead-Allwood, had to cut it in two places. My scar went from the hip to the knee. But eventually she sorted it out, and I was on the road to recovery.

Soon after discharge, however, I suffered severe abdominal pain. Sheelagh called an ambulance, because we were not absolutely sure whether the pain was abdominal or cardiac. The ambulance men did a quick ECG check, and when I looked at it I was reassured. They took me to the Whittington Hospital where they diagnosed a cholecystitis (inflammation of the gall bladder). I was not happy with the diagnosis, suspecting gallstones, so after discharge we arranged for a private MRI scan. My gall bladder was full of stones, which had not been detected at the Whittington. About a month later I had to have a laparoscopic cholecystectomy. I was told that I would

213

be in hospital for a day or two. After the operation I felt great, but during the first post-operative night I suffered a bad bout of pain. I called the nurses, but no one came. After thirty minutes or so, with some hesitation, I dialled the mobile number of my surgeon, as he had told me to contact him at any time if I had a problem. It was 3 a.m., and he came in half an hour. He tried to contact the nurses while driving, but he, too, had no luck. He thought my problem was some sand in the bile duct, and the pain eventually subsided after medication. Unfortunately I continued to drain bile. The surgeon told me that I probably had an accessory duct of Luschke, which they often do not spot during surgery, as it is hard to detect. But he reassured me that the drainage would stop in a few days.

I experienced another episode of bad pain, so eventually they decided to perform gastroscopy and cut the sphincter in Vater's papilla. Instead of twenty-four hours I spent twelve days in the hospital. Sheelagh had previously told me I was a real sucker for surgery and at the first sign of a problem I would choose to have an operation. She went on to say that up till then I had been lucky, as everything had gone fine, but that sooner or later I would encounter a problem. As she had made this prediction shortly before my surgery I blamed her for jinxing my post-operative recovery.

In September I went again to Bergamo, and then Sheelagh and I went for two weeks to Mandelieu. I also attended the annual meting of the EACTS in Vienna. By now I was not attending the scientific sessions; we just went to see friends at the past presidents' dinner, the wine tasting, the presidential dinner and the presidential reception, which was given after the current president had delivered his address. We had a delightful excursion on the Danube, visited Melk Abbey and went to the opera. To finish my 'medical year' I had my left hip replaced in December.

At the beginning of 2010 I was visiting Jaroslav in the care home every other day. Kate was absolutely wonderful and Daniel very supportive. I thought that for his age he was amazing, joking with his father even when he seemed so ill. One day I was driving to Acton and the traffic on the A406 was moving at a snail's pace. I must have dozed off, as suddenly I felt a jolt. I had gone into the car ahead of me. There was not much damage, but when I was driving home after seeing Jaroslav water started leaking from the cooling system. I had to stop at a petrol station and call the AA. After a two-hour wait they towed me to a garage to get the leak repaired.

My hip surgeon Sarah allowed me to play golf once more at the end of February. On Saturday the 20th I was practising pitching on the fifth fairway next to her. I finished first and went back to the clubhouse. I was cleaning my shoes with a high-pressure air hose when I twisted my foot, thus dislocating my operated hip. Sarah and Sheelagh called an ambulance, but there was a problem. As the NHS ambulance could not take me to the Princess Grace, a private hospital, they tried unsuccessfully to summon a private ambulance. Eventually Sarah was able to persuade the NHS ambulance to take me there. I was in real agony before the ambulance arrived, lying on the tarmac in the car park. It started snowing, and a kind lady member stood above me holding an umbrella. The ambulance drove to the Princess Grace via the Holloway Road; it was match day at the Arsenal Stadium, and the road was completely blocked. It took them about an hour to reach the hospital where I was taken straight to theatre. Fortunately Sarah was able to put the hip back under anaesthesia without opening me up. I recovered well, and by March I was playing golf again. In May I went to Bergamo for the last time.

In July we took Kate and Daniel to a cottage in Dorset for a break. They seemed to be coping in the aftermath of Jaroslav's death – Daniel perhaps better than Kate, who became very low in mood a few months later; she did not shake off severe depression for a year and a half.

In September Sheelagh and I went to the EACTS meeting in Geneva and visited Michael and Joan Deeny again in Anzère. In October we had three weeks in Mandelieu, being joined for a week by Květa and Peter Trent from Highgate Golf Club. Finally, in November, we went with the Chaumetons to Paris to see a Monet exhibition in the Petit Palais. I tried to organize the trip myself, but having arranged what I thought was a good price for the Eurostar train and the hotel I then called Tim, our travel agent in Bath. He found a good three-star hotel with the train journey included in the price, which was a much better deal. While in Paris we went to the Musée d'Art Moderne, to the Trocadero and to an exhibition about the Medici family; it was a highly cultural trip. After our return Sheelagh and I had a week in New York seeing three plays, visiting the Museum of Modern Art, the Metropolitan Museum and the Frick Collection. We also had a lunch with an old friend, Dr Jan Quagebauer, who was chief of congenital heart surgery at Columbia University, and we had an excellent time. We spent Christmas in Mandelieu and enjoyed a Christmas Eve dinner in the Colombe d'Or in St Paul de Vence. Early in 2011 I had a tooth implant in Prague. I went there three times, but even including the airfares the total cost was about a third of the cost quoted in London. My friend Honza Marek highly recommended Docent Urban, who did an excellent good job.

In February and March Sheelagh and I had a long holiday in New Zealand. We flew to Japan, visiting Kyoto and Nara. I had been there some years ago, so I wrote to Dr Shigehito Miki asking if one of his staff could show us around and offering to give them a lecture in return. In Kyoto we stayed in a *ryokan*, a typical Japanese bed-and-breakfast establishment. We were intrigued to note that of all the people staying there we were the only ones who asked for a Japanese breakfast. At the entrance to the house we had to change into slippers and then into a different pair of slippers before entering our room. A pretty Japanese girl in a stylish kimono served us our breakfast, which consisted of ten dishes. At nighttime they moved the little table aside and spread mattresses and blankets on the floor. It was very cold outside, but we had an efficient heater in the room. The main drawback was the bathroom, which was tiny and freezing.

We took a look around Kyoto, and then the paediatric cardiac surgeon and the deputy director of the hospital from Nara collected us. During the drive it started to snow heavily. We visited the famous Nara Park with its deer and several remarkable Buddhist temples, and the deer tried to pick food from our pockets. The deputy director was wearing flip-flops, so it was hard for him to walk in the snow, and the drive to Nara hospital proved impossible, as the traffic had come to a complete halt in the snowstorm. In addition, the chief surgeon at the hospital was taken ill with kidney stones. They therefore decided to cancel my lecture.

We were able to drive to a restaurant where they had booked a traditional Japanese banquet. I met Dr Miki and Dr Kenji Kusuhara again. Dr Miki was in London with Donald Ross for about eight years, and Dr Kusuhara had been with us at Great Ormond Street for a year with his wife. It was a lovely reunion. Sheelagh and I were wearing fairly formal dress for my lecture and the banquet, but most of the doctors turned up in jeans and without ties. Next day we returned to Tokyo on the bullet train and went straight to the airport. On the way we saw snow-capped Mount Fuji in the distance.

From Japan we flew via Sydney to Auckland. In Sydney we had some time to kill, but fortunately we were in the airport business lounge. So we had a shower and a good breakfast, and the time passed easily. In Auckland we met Sheelagh's relative Hugh McArdle, a radiologist, who showed us around. In the evening we went for dinner with his Chinese girlfriend at the revolving tower restaurant, from where we had wonderful views over the city. The next day we hired a car and drove north. The first stop was Waitomo Lodge. The owners were friendly people, and there was a pool on the deck with a Jacuzzi. Each evening we had cake left by our hosts in the fridge. The views over the bay were phenomenal, and we had a memorable boat trip around the Bay of a Thousand Islands.

We also met Irenka Trnka and her husband Ben, who had bought a summer-house on the northern tip of the North Island, as Irenka's sister lived in Auckland. We played golf with them and visited their home. We then left our hire car at the airport in Kerikeri and flew to Lake Taupo where we stayed in a lovely place, Acacia Lodge, which was beautifully decorated. The views over Lake Taupo were impressive, and we enjoyed excellent food with our hosts, who were young and charming, on their deck with the other guests in the evenings. The husband was a professional chef, and his meals were of a very high standard. We played golf at Waikerie, a championship course, which was beautiful. We also visited Rotarua's hot springs and geysers.

A disastrous earthquake in Christchurch struck while we were on the North Island; fortunately we were not affected, and we merely followed the news on TV. We hired a car once more in Taupo and drove south to Hastings, where we played some golf and had a memorable trip on the trailer of a tractor that drove under the cliffs so that we could see all the geology, remnants of earthquakes as well as a colony of gannets. This was located near Cape Kidnappers where our friends Maureen and Toni had stayed the previous year.

Our golfing experiences in New Zealand were mixed but overall pleasant. Some golf courses had only a wooden hut as a clubhouse, and we found it was often locked. In front of one hut we saw a notice saying, 'Put $20 in the box and play', which we thought was great.

Afterwards we went to Wellington, where we stayed with Anne Harden who used to work at Great Ormond Street in the EEG Department. First we visited her niece on their farm north of Wellington and played golf with her husband. The farm was enormous; they took us for a drive, and as far as the eye could see it was their land. Everything was highly automated, and just two people looked after 400 cows – which included milking them. Anne showed us around Wellington, where had three really good days. At eighty-one years of age she was still adventurous and energetic. She travelled abroad frequently on her own and managed a large house and extensive garden, which she kept beautifully, and she entertained us admirably the entire time we were there.

The last day we took a ferry to the South Island, which took about four hours, and drove to the Marlborough region. We played golf at Oyster Bay, then tasted wine at Saint Clair and at Scott's, another winery. We had several excellent meals in wineries, where the steaks were succulent and tender. Sheelagh commented every time she ate one that it was the best she had ever eaten. But in the next winery down the road she thought the steaks were even better! From Marlborough we drove to Nelson where we stayed at a B&B run by two gay men. It was interestingly furnished, and they were slightly bohemian and great company. Moreover the house had superb views over the sea. We made a one-day boat trip to the Tasman National Park and went for a long walk. From Nelson we followed the west coast of the South Island to Punakaiki where there were jewellery shops selling mainly jade. There was very interesting geology to be viewed there, with pancake rocks and blow holes and other unusual rock formations. We had never seen anything like it before. Franz Josef and Fox Glaciers were worth visiting and, of course, Lake Matheson, which is said to be the most photographed lake in New Zealand.

While driving south through the Haast Pass we were almost eaten alive by sandflies. We had been warned previously about them, but there was little we could do to protect ourselves. We continued to Lake Wanaka and to Arrowtown, where we stayed in a very pleasant B&B recommended by our friends the Slaters. The couple who owned it were somewhat eccentric but kindly and jovial and left homemade bread and cake in our room each day. They insisted on our joining them for a drink every evening so that they could enjoy hearing about our experiences.

We then visited Queenstown, where we took a cable car to the top of the mountain for some remarkable views before driving further south. We played golf at Lake Te Anau and had delicious venison that evening and then continued to embark on a boat for a 24-hour cruise on Doubtful Sound. This

HOUSE RENOVATIONS AND FURTHER HOLIDAYS, 2008–2015

was the experience of a lifetime, travelling through the fjords late in the evening with the sunset and again in the early misty morning – albeit with the sandflies still biting. At this time there was a second devastating earthquake in Japan, in Fukushima, but no tsunami approached. Lake Tekapo's golf course is the highest in altitude in New Zealand. We decided to avoid Christchurch because of the recent earthquake and drove directly to the airport on its outskirts, where we returned our car and flew to Hawaii.

There Sheelagh and I stayed in a comfortable bungalow at Ke Iki Hale on the north shore of the Big Island, where I had stayed some years ago after the World Congress of Paediatric Cardiology in Honolulu. There were gigantic waves, and we watched remarkably skilled surfers battling the elements. We played some golf, drove around the island and generally had a good time. From Hawaii we flew to San Francisco where we stayed for a couple of days and visited Bob Szarnicki and his wife Mary. Mary is of Irish descent, and as it was St Patrick's Day we had a wonderful Irish–American meal and celebration. Their children, aged around twenty-three and twenty-seven, joined us later.

Our final stop was to visit Sheelagh's sister Bronagh and her family in Portland, Oregon, before flying back to London.

In May, June and September we had our usual two weeks in Mandelieu, and in August I took Daniel to Prague and Senohraby. He developed *Herpes zoster* the day after our arrival but managed to enjoy himself anyway. Jiřina, my sister's daughter, and Ládík, her husband, took him on a couple of enjoyable trips. Later on Sheelagh and I went to Baltimore near Cork to Oliver's and Cecilia's wedding anniversary. There was a gathering of about fifty members of the Woods family who had come from all parts of the globe to Ireland to celebrate, including Oliver's seven children and their families, and it was a very lively occasion.

In November we were invited once more by the Newmans to Barbados. The golf was excellent, and overall it was very good fun. We spent Christmas in Mandelieu, where we experienced fine weather and had an enjoyable time. For Christmas Eve dinner we went to the Colombe d'Or restaurant in St Paul de Vence, but this time we booked a room and stayed overnight to avoid driving back to our flat at the end of the evening. Before dinner we went for a walk with the idea of having a drink somewhere in the village. But no – on Christmas Eve everything is closed in France; it is a family holiday, so nothing is open. Eventually we found a little wine shop in a cellar. A young man there was very pleasant and sold us a half-bottle of white and a bottle of red wine, which we drank in the hotel room. The menu in the restaurant was very good, and we gleaned some enjoyment watching the other guests. A Russian couple was sitting at the next table; the woman ordered a single glass of red wine, which she nursed the whole evening, while her companion ordered one vodka after another, which he mostly drank neat. During the holidays we had exceptionally fine weather, which was a bonus, and we spent quite a bit of time with an English friend living in Cannes, Nick Kent.

In February and March 2012 we continued our series of long holidays. We went to Thailand, Laos, Vietnam, Cambodia and Thailand over the course of almost six weeks. We started in Bangkok, staying at the Mandarin Oriental Hotel. Our travel agent had told us it was a must. There were superb orchids in the foyer, a lovely swimming-pool, and we experienced great service. My old friend Pantpis Sakornpant and his English wife Clare took us for a day's outing to Ayutthaya, the ancient capital of Siam which I had visited some years earlier with Jaroslav and Kate. The one problem with our outing was that Pantpis had hired a professional guide, who he plainly did not need, as he kept correcting her facts, which was very embarrassing. Clare was not happy about her husband's interventions – but he was unstoppable. At any rate we had a very good day. From Bangkok we flew to Chiang Mai, where we visited an orchid farm and an elephant training school. We bought a picture painted by an elephant; we actually watched the elephants painting and discovered that they could be trained to do all sorts of things, including playing football and basketball and generally amusing visitors by pulling off their hats, accepting tips and so on. We played golf accompanied by female caddies.

The next stop was Chiang Rai, where we visited the local market. This was extraordinarily interesting and colourful and gave us a real taste of local life. On the way there our guide stopped for lunch in an excellent restaurant called Cabbages and Condoms. They had an ongoing campaign against HIV and Aids, with all the profits from the restaurant going to this cause. The food there was delicious.

After Chiang Rai we were taken by car to the Mekong River and spent two days on a boat travelling down to Laos. As we cruised along we saw many local villages with children selling embroidered bracelets they had made themselves. They were very reluctant to let you go, and one little girl actually followed Sheelagh back to the boat – Sheelagh felt so sorry for the child that she gave her some money. There was evidently great poverty there; the majority of the children looked small for their age, presumably owing to malnutrition. One night we stayed in a lodge where the children from the village near by organized a musical evening for us, dancing, singing and playing instruments.

We disembarked in Luang Prabang, the second largest city in Laos. Our guide, a highly educated and intelligent man, told us that life had been bad under Communism but now it had greatly improved. When I mentioned that they were still a Communist state he replied that this was true but that the purpose of the Communist Party was to ensure that the transition to capitalism was smooth. The temples were fascinating, as they had walls of mosaics depicting historical events. The street markets were vibrant, and the waterfalls highly picturesque. I even had a swim there. We also saw some bears in a sanctuary. We made the mistake of eating some eggs injected with a coriander mixture from a street stall, and this was to have a bad effect on our digestive tracts, especially Sheelagh's, but fortunately she recovered within twenty-four hours. After this we visited a gallery run by a French woman and a Swiss man dedicated to the promotion of Laotian artists; they displayed some interesting paintings but mainly beautiful textiles. We explored the local temples; some had wonderful mosaics depicting ancient myths on their walls. We also saw large pallets of flatbread being dried in the sun.

We celebrated Sheelagh's birthday in Laos. Her cousin Christina, one of the managing directors of the Orient Express chain of hotels, knew the manager of the best hotel and restaurant in Luang Prabang and had told him of our visit. After our arrival I phoned the hotel, called La Résidence. The manager was extraordinarily helpful; he sent a car for us in the evening, and we had a wonderful meal by the beautifully lit hotel pool – and he charged us half-price. Our guide later told us that he had been engaged and had been saving up money to pay for ten pigs he was supposed to give to the parents of the bride. But just before the wedding a Laotian from the same tribe, who was living in California, came home for a visit. He took a shine to the girl and bought her from her parents, and that was that. The guide explained to us that the life of juvenile brides taken off to the USA was not always a happy one. Their husbands would often lock them up in the morning and go off to work all day, so that the girls were practically slaves in the house.

From Luang Prabang we flew to Hanoi, where we saw the water-puppet theatre, ate some good meals and each had a massage. Sheelagh had asked for a firm massage, but after a few minutes she changed her request to a light one, as she didn't want to end up covered in bruises! Watching street life was a novelty. Generally there are no traffic lights; vehicles come eight abreast from every direction, with some motorbikes carrying a full load of pigs or chickens on the back, and they all have to negotiate roundabouts and crossings. Remarkably we did not witness any accidents. Our guide explained to us that in Vietnam they did not have VIPs, only CIPs (Communist Important Persons). People in general smiled a lot and seemed happy enough. But we heard that there was still considerable poverty – and a great deal of bribery and corruption. The presidential palace, which was now a museum, was an interesting site, as was the military museum, although the barbed-wire cages used for solitary confinement were horrific. The Maison Central was the main prison used originally by the French, later to imprison Communists and finally to house American pilots shot down during the Vietnam War. They had a guillotine in one room, and we were informed that it had been used until quite recently. Meanwhile our hotel in the middle of the old French quarter in Hanoi was extremely comfortable.

From Hanoi we were driven to Halong Bay, which was about three hours' journey. We boarded a boat there and settled into a luxury cabin with a terrace and a Jacuzzi. Halong Bay has around 2,900 islands and rock formations jutting out of the sea. We saw a floating village and some incredible rocks. It was photographer's paradise, especially in the morning mist, which made the scene especially romantic. The boat trip was highly memorable, as was a visit to one of the islands. We set off on bicycles, but I had not been on one for around sixty years, and they were designed for small Vietnamese people, which made pedalling difficult for an average-sized Westerner. But eventually I mastered my bike – to the amazement of our guide.

The next stop was Hue, a former city of the kings. Its citadel, palaces and pyramids were fascinating. We walked through it, visited the local market and had a delicious evening meal at the Hotel Résidence, where we stayed. From Hue we drove to Denang, which had been used as a rest-and-recreation place for US troops during the Vietnam War. The beaches there were extensive, with fine white sand. We visited an interesting ethnic museum and went to a mountain with a marble factory with some very beautiful traditional and modern sculptures. During the Vietnam War there had been a Vietcong field hospital inside the caves in the marble mountain.

We then drove to Hoi An, a small town with around 200 tailors, 150 shoemakers and the same number of opticians. We had some spectacles made up, and I had trousers and two shirts tailored, while Sheelagh had a trouser suit and a skirt made from silk we bought in Thailand.

The first day our guide took us to his friend's restaurant for a delicious lunch. The next day we went to the local village, where they showed us how to prepare an area of ground for planting vegetables and how to fertilize them and water them with cans connected to one another by a long wooden pole supported over the shoulders; one rotated the cans with each hand. We also took an afternoon course in Vietnamese cooking at the Red Bridge Cookery School.

From Hoi An we flew to Saigon or Ho Chi Minh City, as it is now known. Our guide there was a very pleasant and knowledgeable man. We visited the Roman Catholic Notre Dame cathedral and the main Post Office, which was designed by the same architect as the Eiffel Tower. Our guide took us also to a multi-denominational church, which was used by Catholics one day, Protestants the next and by Jews the day after that. We also visited the famous Cu Chi tunnels outside Saigon. The construction of these was started by the French, but they were enlarged by the Vietcong. There were about 250 kilometres of tunnels at three different levels, at depths of three, six and ten metres. The entrances were small, and only a slim Vietnamese person could pass through. When they entered they concealed the hole with a wooden cover masked by grass and leaves so no one would guess that anything was beneath. The air vents from the kitchens looked like termite nests. One could walk right past and not realize a thing. When the Americans erected their camps they were surprised that so many of their men were shot in their tents during the night by the Vietcong, but they had constructed some of their camps above the tunnels.

From Saigon we drove to the Mekong river delta, which has nine channels flowing into the sea. It is one of the world's longest rivers, originating on the Tibetan plateau and flowing between Burma and Laos, along the border between Laos and Thailand, down to Cambodia and Vietnam. We spent two days and a night on the boat, saw a floating market, watched the life on the river and visited a village. Finally we took a boat to Chau Doc, where we spent a night and then went on to Phnom Penh, the capital of Cambodia. The Royal Palace, Silver Pagoda and National Museum took some time to explore. We also went to see the Killing Fields, left as a lasting memorial to the terrible legacy of the Khmer Rouge and Pol Pot. We could not understand why he had not been tried after the fall of his regime, as the atrocities he had committed were so appalling. We were told that he had been exiled to a remote region where he died in a small hut.

At this point we felt we needed some respite from the gruelling recent history of the country, and the market in Phnom Penh with its deep-fried insects and peeled frogs was well worth a visit. There we were especially intrigued by the tradition of putting a snake in each whisky bottle.

The highlight of Cambodia was certainly Siem Reap with Angkor Wat. It was an incredible sight considering that most of the temples had been constructed between the ninth and twelfth centuries. Some of the decorations and statues had been designed originally in the Buddhist fashion, but later, when the regime changed, they were altered to appear more Hindu in style. We had to get up early to see the sunrise, which meant being there before 5 a.m., but it was well worth it. We were advised to take a packed breakfast from the hotel, so when all the tourists returned to their hotels for breakfast we had a swift picnic meal and enjoyed the ruins without being surrounded by hordes of other foreigners. Beng Mealen was a very impressive and beautiful temple almost completely obscured by jungle vegetation, and some of the pictures I took there are spectacular.

From Siem Reap we took a plane to Phuket via Bangkok. Our plan was to relax after more then four weeks of hard travelling. Christina, Sheelagh's cousin, recommended the Banyan Tree, where instead of rooms each couple had a secluded villa with its own swimming-pool. It was blissful. Coming back hot and sticky from the nearby golf course and jumping into the pool was a great treat. The garden walls were high, so in the morning one could jump into one's pool stark naked without fear of being overlooked. You were taken anywhere you wanted to go by golf buggy. The beach was about 100 metres away, so we usually went to the small coastal restaurants good and cheap meals washed down with a bottle of wine. The only down side was the presence of many overweight and noisy Russians.

HOUSE RENOVATIONS AND FURTHER HOLIDAYS, 2008–2015

In May, June and September we went to Mandelieu as usual, and in July we visited Oliver and Cecilia in Armagh. In October we went to the annual EACTS meeting in Barcelona, where we stayed in the Casa Fuster, a lovely hotel recommended by our friend Mo Murtra. It was away from the hustle of the meeting and was centrally located. We spent some time in the Picasso museum and at the Miró Foundation. A tapas bar called Cerveceria Catalunya, recommended by the doorman in our hotel, was particularly good. One could sit at the bar, order wine or beer and point to the tapas one fancied, all of which were delicious and good value. The presidential dinner was held in Montjuïc, which reminded me of the time when I was the association's president, as it was in exactly the same place. As the building is a museum of Catalan art we were able to see some of the exhibits before dinner, including many beautiful medieval frescoes, pictures and statues. During the dinner there was a wonderful exhibition of Flamenco-dancing. One couple danced on a platform in each corner of the hall.

In December I visited my sister in Prague. Christmas was once more spent in Mandelieu and consisted of plenty of golf and Christmas dinner with our English friend Nick in Gaston et Gastounette in Cannes.

The year 2013 started with another great holiday, this time to Mexico and Guatemala, although our flight to Mexico City was not without problems. The day of our departure it started snowing, so we were delayed for about four hours because all the aircrafts had to be de-iced. In Mexico City we spent the next half-day in the fascinating Museum of Anthropology. Our guide Mario was well informed and a great individual. We went to the Palacio Nacional to see the murals of Diego Rivera, then on to the cathedral. In front we saw a beautifully dressed young girl and were told that she was going to a coming-of-age ceremony traditionally held at sixteen years. Sheelagh thought that she looked older, but I had a picture taken with her anyway. Our next day was free, so we went to see the Frida Kahlo Museum and her house and also the studio of Diego Rivera. Kahlo's house was extremely colourful, while Rivera's was a large black stone building where he collected Mayan artefacts. He had amassed a collection of about 30,000 pieces, which, before he died, he gave to the nation. Frida Kahlo married and divorced Rivera twice and was the mistress of Trotsky, who lived for some time in their house.

In Mexico City we ventured on to the underground train system. On our return Lorcan, Sheelagh's nephew, who had worked in Mexico for three years, told us that it was a crazy and dangerous thing to do unaccompanied. Even he had never done that – and his name means 'fierce little one' in Irish. But in our ignorance we felt safe, as we had been shown the ropes the first day by our guide. The next d ay we were accompanied to Teotihuacan to see the Pyramids of the Moon and the Sun. On the way back we stopped at the modern Cathedral of Nuestra Señora de Guadalupe, which was a very impressive building holding up to 8,000 people; the previous year it had been visited by 8.5 million people between 9 and 12 December, important dates in the Mayan calendar. The old Baroque church was splitting into two because of subsidence; when I showed friends my photographs they thought I had tilted the camera.

The fourth day we flew to Villahermosa. Our flight was delayed, so we did not have time to go to La Venta, where they have a collection of square Olmec heads. We were taken straight to Palenque, one of the most important Mayan sites. After about two hours at the site it started raining, and within a few minutes it had turned into a real downpour. Having waited for about half an hour we asked our guide, who was wearing a waterproof jacket, if he would fetch us some waterproofs being sold at the entrance to the site. He duly bought them for us, so we made it to the car in a reasonably dry state. That night we stayed in a comfortable bungalow near the Palenque site. It was in the jungle, so everything was very humid. Nothing would dry overnight. We put our shoes outside hoping that they would dry better there. In the morning, when I opened the door to collect them, a large black bird flew into our room, and it took some effort to get him out. The next day we visited La Venta, which had some unusual animals in its zoo. And some of its huge Olmec heads weighed more than twenty tons. They had been transported there from the coast, where they were in danger of being damaged by oil production works.

After visiting Venta Park we flew to Merida, where we stayed in a pleasant hotel in the middle of the city. Around the corner was an excellent restaurant called Chaya, where we tasted the Chaya drink for the first time. I certainly liked it. It is not tea – *chai* – but an alcoholic drink made from the leaves of a local shrub. The next day we went walking about, looking around the cathedral, the municipal house and the Pareo de Montejo, the main street with many lovely buildings. In the evening someone suggested that we visit a genuine Mayan shop. We ended up buying two Panama hats, which were supposed to be better in Merida then in Ecuador. They are made from a material that apparently repels mosquitoes. In the evening we went to a concert on the square near our hotel. They hold one there weekly, and it was certainly worth going. We experienced some great dancing, singing and colourful costumes in the packed square. The next day we visited Uxmal and Kabah, two more Mayan sites. Kabah was particularly memorable, as we arrived with our guide before any other the tourists and had the place to ourselves.

In the morning our guide and driver took us to Chichen Itza, where we stayed overnight. This is a huge site with pyramids as well as a large court for playing a special ball game and a cenote, a natural pool of water where they used to sacrifice young girls. They would drug them with a hallucinogenic drink and then push them into the cenote.

The ball game consisted of getting a ball through a high ring attached to a wall without using hands, feet or head. It sometimes took several days before the first goal was scored. At the end of the game the captain of the winning team was beheaded as a sacrifice – apparently the greatest possible honour. Chichen Itza is a magnificent site unfortunately spoiled by too many tourists and vendors. From there we drove to Cancún, where we had the rest of the day to relax. The hotel had a fantastic beach and beautiful views along the coast. In the evening we went to a traditional seafood restaurant, with a great atmosphere and fantastic food.

In the morning we flew via San Salvador to Guatemala City. We were somewhat taken aback at the boarding gate in San Salvador to see the weather forecast for Guatemala City, which was –8 degrees centigrade. Fortunately it was 22 degrees by the time we landed there.

From the airport our driver took us straight to Antigua, an attractive small town surrounded by three volcanoes. It was destroyed by a volcanic eruption around 1780 and became a ghost town for about a hundred years. It is now much restored and very beautiful. Some ruins of churches and monasteries were impressive. We stayed at the Posada Don Rodrigo with patios full of shrubs and flowers. Mariachi music was played in the evening during dinner.

The next day we walked through the town seeing all the sights: the cathedral, the municipal Palacio and numerous monasteries, churches and fountains. We found the Convento San Domenico especially fascinating.

They had six museums, a large lecture hall and lovely gardens where we had a candlelit dinner. From Antigua we drove to Lake Atitlán, the third largest lake in Guatemala. On the way we stopped in San Juan Comalpo, where we went to a local school and talked to some of the children. We photographed them and some of the colourful murals on the wall along the main road painted by the local youth. The cemetery was also highly interesting. There were elaborate tombs, since everyone was keen to have a nice 'last house'. Afterwards we visited the market, which was vibrant and busy with butchers, vegetable and fruit stalls, textiles, shoe polishing and much more.

We arrived at Lake Atitlán in the late afternoon. Hotel Atitlán was beautifully furnished with antique furniture and surrounded by huge grounds full of lovely trees, flowers and birds including colourful parrots. We had a special dinner in the hotel to celebrate my birthday. The next day there we went on an excursion to Panajachel and took a boat across the lake to Santiago. We saw a local hospital, which was minuscule but apparently well run. The two consulting-rooms looked, from the outside, like a pair of toilets. After lunch on the shore of the lake we drove to Chichicastanego, famous for its market and cathedral. In the latter they have a mass conducted by the Catholic priest one day and the next day a celebration of Mayan customs by a shaman. Sometimes both officiate at the same time. We stayed in the Hotel San Tommaso with many patios and much religious regalia; in our room there was a full set of priest's garments on the wall.

Next day we drove to Guatemala City. Our driver's car had a problem, as the passenger window would not close. Fortunately the driver managed to obtain some plastic sheeting, which he secured over the window to shelter us from the elements. It was cold and rainy and we were about 2,200 metres above sea level. After we arrived in Guatemala City I called Aldo Castaneda to confirm our golfing arrangements for the next day. Aldo had an interesting life story. He was Guatemalan but born in Italy. He spent the Second World War in Germany, where his grandfather was an ambassador. After the war he studied medicine in Guatemala City and then went to the USA for postgraduate training. He trained mainly with Dr Richard Varco in Minneapolis, and when Dr Varco accidentally cut his wrist tendons and median nerve Aldo started doing all the surgery there. He was eventually appointed chief of congenital heart surgery at Boston Children's Hospital. So his story was not so dissimilar to mine, and we hit it off from our very

HOUSE RENOVATIONS AND FURTHER HOLIDAYS, 2008–2015

first meeting. He had moved back to Guatemala City for his retirement. When we met he took us to his golf club, which was very special, as there were not many people around. We had a very enjoyable round in the morning and a good opportunity to talk and catch up. After lunch he showed us the hospital he had built. He had organized a congenital cardiac unit for poor children, raising money both in the USA and in Guatemala. He had worked without a salary in the hospital for the past thirteen years since his retirement from Boston Children's Hospital. The hospital was very well equipped, and we visited the wards, the intensive care unit and the catheterization laboratory. Aldo went to the hospital every morning at 7 to do the ward round. Then he would assists the surgeons he had trained with various operations, and if it was something particularly difficult he would perform it himself. Remarkably he is now approaching his mid-eighties.

In the evening we had dinner at his and his wife's apartment, in an unusual round building where they have the whole of the sixth floor to themselves; more usually there are four flats on one floor. The apartment was beautifully furnished with magnificent carpets, pictures and sculptures. Aldo surprised us. Our guide for the past four days had told us a great deal about the history of the country, about the thirty years of bloody civil war. But now, he said, the country was safe. Aldo took a completely different view. His three children and all his grandchildren live in the USA, and he does not allow them to visit him in Guatemala because he considers it too dangerous. He said that the newspapers had reported twenty homicides during the previous weekend. And there was a danger of kidnapping, too. Sheelagh and I were somewhat taken aback, as we had walked around freely at all times of the day and night. Aldo's building had metal entry gates into the grounds, and there was a double lock to get into the building. His floor could be accessed only with a special key in the lift. It was powerfully secured.

From Guatemala City we flew to Flores to visit Tikal, the most impressive Mayan site in Guatemala. It is 500 kilometres square, and only a small part has been discovered and opened up to visitors. We stayed about 30 kilometres away in a bungalow by a lake. It was a lovely open place with around eight bungalows on several levels above the lake, not at all encroaching on each other. We had our meals upstairs where they had a bar and tables surrounded by trees. One evening an owl came to visit us in the rafters. In the afternoon we went down to the lake, which took some effort as the path was very steep. By the lake were two canoes, so we borrowed one and went paddling. After lunch a group of six English people invited us to go with them on a speedboat to Flores, about an hour's ride across the lake. It is the regional capital with some very interesting architecture. We happily accepted the invitation and had a very pleasant afternoon with them. Before we boarded the boat to return it started raining heavily. Sheelagh and I sheltered in a little bar, but during the ride back everyone got soaked, although we had our anoraks on so remained relatively dry. The following day we visited Tikal, which was most impressive. Our guide, of Italian extraction, was very witty and well informed. The Mayan remnants and the jungle were unforgettable. Altogether we spent a most enjoyable three days in the area.

To get from Flores to Cancún was not easy. Although Cancún is due north, only about 500 kilometres from Flores, we had to fly back to Guatemala City and from there to Mexico City, which was a huge detour, and only then from Mexico City to Cancún. We were not advised about the time change, so we had just two hours to change planes in Mexico City. We were informed that this was not long enough but decided to risk it. When we came to the immigration hall at Mexico City Airport we realized that it was a real problem. About a hundred people were ahead of us in the queue, which was moving at a snail's pace. I suggested to Sheelagh that she go to the head of the queue to explain our situation and see if someone would let us through. It worked, so a few minutes later I joined her. The nice man who let us through was half-Czech and planning to visit the Czech Republic, so I gave him my email address and promised to help with the planning of his trip.

We successfully made the plane and arrived in Cancun at 8 p.m. From the airport we were taken to Secrets Capri, a delightful hotel in Playa del Carmen, about 45 kilometres south. The Chaumetons, our golfing and bridge partners, were waiting for us there. The hotel had a lovely sandy beach and three swimming-pools. It was a hotel with an all-inclusive package, so one was spoiled for choice. There were five restaurants, several bars and the only problem was deciding what to have for one's first, then second and then third drink. It was also tricky to decide whether to go for Japanese, Italian, Mexican, seafood or American food. Apart from relaxing we played bridge together and had three rounds of golf. So altogether it was a very successful holiday.

Soon after we arrived home we went for a five-day break to Florence. I had pre-booked tickets for the Uffizi Gallery, the Palatine Gallery in the Pitti Palace and the Bargello Museum. Anne Chaumeton was not especially happy about this, as she would have preferred to do things spontaneously. But when we reached the museums I think she appreciated my booking in advance, since there were huge queues for tickets, whereas we walked straight in. A similar situation occurred with the booking of our evening meals. I had asked two or three of my Italian cardiac surgeon friends for recommendations and booked three dinners in advance. I felt that we could always cancel but that without booking it might be difficult to get into the best restaurants. One never knew in Florence; it was such a popular tourist destination.

In March I visited Prague, while Sheelagh went back to Mexico to join her sister Bronagh and her family for her sister's seventy-fifth birthday. In April, May and June we went as usual to Mandelieu. In July I took Daniel to Prague, and in August Sheelagh and I went to Belgium to stay with Marc and Vicki de Leval. In September we were back in Mandelieu, and Oliver and Cecilia came to join us for a week. The EACTS meeting that year was held in Barcelona, and I duly attended this.

The highlight of the year was our trip to the Antarctic. I had wanted to go for some time, but it was only now that we could do so. It exceeded all our expectations. On 1 December we flew from London via Buenos Aires to Ushuaia, the most southerly town in Argentina. On the pier they had a noticeboard saying '*Fin del Mundo*' – the end of the world. We were taken to a good hotel on the shore of a lake where we had lunch with Max, a convivial Dane. It was his fifth trip to the polar regions. The next day in the afternoon we boarded our ship and had our first briefing. The team was impressive. Cheli was a New Zealand woman, around 1.8 metres tall, a no-nonsense individual and a great leader. All the others were experts in their fields, such as icebergs, penguins, whales, birds, the history of the region, its geology and so on. On board we met some kindred spirits, including a couple from Arizona; the wife was originally from Australia. They were very much into flying, as they owned two planes and lived next to an airport. Altogether there were about a hundred passengers and ninety crew. They accepted some youngsters, backpackers and others as last-minute late bookings, which brought the average age well down.

When we left Ushuaia a severe storm was forecast, so the captain decided to shelter for twenty-four hours behind the nearby island. We experienced a swell of around three metres, but on the other side it was more like twelve to fifteen. The captain had made a good decision. While sailing to South Georgia we had three to four lectures each day. They called the days E&E Days (Eating and Education). We had talks about ice in the Antarctic, on the whales of the Southern Ocean, Shackleton's Antarctic adventures and various other topics. It was all fascinating stuff. The next day in the afternoon we saw several killer whales. South Georgia was a paradise for wildlife. They call it the Galapagos of the Antarctic. When we had the first landing we saw a large colony of penguins. I asked the guide how many were there. He said to count the legs and divide by two! But then he added that there were probably about 450,000 penguins. We had several landings in Zodiac inflatable boats every day. As they gave us warm anoraks we were very comfortable. In Stromness we saw the remnants of the whaling station that Shackleton, Worsley and Green had reached after their epic boat journey from Elephant Island from where they walked across the mountains. We saw king penguins and later on Adélie and chinstraps, which were all fascinating to observe. The couples share parental duties sitting on the eggs. When one goes fishing, sometimes several kilometres away, on returning the bird finds its partner by the sound of its cry within the large colony.

We had a small disaster in our cabin. I had forgotten to turn off the water tap in the bathroom when handwashing a few clothes, and when we came back from dinner we found the cabin flooded. Fortunately the domestic staff were able to clear it up.

The elephant seals and fur seals were interesting to watch and photograph. They throw sand over themselves to keep cool. Meanwhile the penguins cool themselves by standing in pools of water. We also saw a leopard seal – a very fascinating creature. We had a couple of parties on the boat, one on a theme of 'Leaving South Georgia', the other on the theme of 'Hats', where everyone showed great initiative and produced the most inventive headgear or costumes out of everyday objects. On landing the next day we saw a large colony of penguins, some of which were moulting, which looked very comical. There was a large number of brown furry young chicks and courting couples close together demonstrating almost human signs of tenderness. In the evening Damien, one of the guides, gave us a talk on how he had been trapped on South Georgia Island during the Falklands conflict.

Our next stop was Elephant Island, where we saw three minor calvings of the glacier, which means that a portion of the glacier splits off from the main part causing tsunamis depending on its size. It was also the first time we saw macaroni penguins with their sticks of spaghetti in different orange colours as a headdress. In the evening we watched the film *Keiko: The Real Story of Ocean Orca from Free Willy*. It was about a killer whale who had been kept in captivity for some years. A group of enthusiasts, sponsored by a very wealthy man, decided to attempt to rehabilitate him so that he could go back into the wild. It was some story. One of our guides was personally involved in the project.

We later visited St Andrew's Bay where we saw a colony of king penguins. Skuas were circling above the colony trying to snatch an egg or a chick. Gentoo penguins also had a colony there. Our next stop was the Antarctic Peninsula, where we saw considerable quantities of pack ice and several minor icebergs. Then came the polar plunge. Participants were put in a harness and encouraged to jump into the ice-cold water at the stern of the ship to be pulled out immediately. Sheelagh and I decided to give that a miss.

The Drake Passage was incredibly calm, not living up to its reputation. On the way back to Ushuaia we passed Cape Horn. We were allowed to come in close to the shore since we had special permission, and it was extremely impressive. After our arrival in Ushuaia we had crab for lunch and then caught our flight to Buenos Aires. After arriving at our hotel we asked where the best place to watch a performance of Argentinian tango might be. We took a taxi to the place recommended by the receptionist, and during dinner we watched a wonderful demonstration of this form of dance. Early the next morning we took a flight to Iguazu near the Iguazu Falls. Christina, Sheelagh's cousin, arranged our stay in the Hotel Los Cataratas. It was a great hotel on the Brazilian side next to the waterfalls located within a national park, so all tourists had to leave by 5 p.m., and they were not allowed to return before 10 a.m. the next day. This offered considerable tranquillity in the evening and early in the morning. The first day we went for a walk along the falls; the next day the taxi took us to the Argentinian side, which was even more impressive than the Brazilian. In the evening we went for dinner and a dance performance in the town of Iguazu. The performance included dancers from Brazil, Paraguay and Argentina, as Iguazu is on the border of all three countries. It was all very skilled. On Saturday, 21 December we caught a flight back to London via Rio de Janeiro. It was undoubtedly one of our most memorable vacations abroad.

We spent Christmas in Mandelieu, returning on New Year's Eve for bridge with the Chaumetons. Then we celebrated my eightieth birthday with a dinner for forty-five people at Highgate Golf Club. During the course of this Gerald Graham and Patrick Ridett gave speeches, as well as Daniel and Kate. At the end of the dinner I announced that we were celebrating not only my birthday but the third anniversary of my marriage to Sheelagh. Our friends were astounded, but the reason we had kept it quiet was simple. We had got married soon after Jaroslav died, so we felt it was not appropriate to celebrate. And as time went by there did not seem to be a suitable opportunity to announce it. However, I did want to tell our friends, so I said to Sheelagh that if we did not announce it at my eightieth the fact would go with us to the grave. Her friends were astounded; they could not believe that she had quiet about our wedding for such a long period of time.

The following week I went to Prague to celebrate my birthday with my family. My sister was equally shocked by the news of our marriage. In February we went for two weeks with Peter and Květa Trent to play golf in South Africa. We had a week in Fancourt and another week in Steenberg, which were both highly enjoyable. Also, because the rate of exchange with the rand was so favourable, it was a cheap holiday. Dinner for four with two bottles of wine cost in the region of £40. In March we accepted an invitation from John and Carol Newman and went for eight days to Barbados. We played a lot of golf at Westmoreland again. I enjoyed the weather, but for Sheelagh it was too hot. In May and June we had two and three weeks respectively in Mandelieu.

In July 2014 Sheelagh and I went to the Czech Republic. After our arrival we had lunch with my sister and then drove in a hired car to Senohraby for coffee and cake and to meet Jiřinka, Tereza and her boyfriend Honzík. We then drove to Třeboň in the south of Bohemia, a wooded area with many huge fish ponds. We did some walking and enjoyed very good Czech cuisine. After three days we drove to Brno, the second largest Czech city. We stayed with Jirka and Hilda Vorlíček, who were wonderful and generous hosts. Jirka had been professor of oncology and later dean of the medical school in Brno. He was one of the first recipients of our Catching Up Fellowships. Meanwhile Hilda had been the head nurse at the Institute of Oncology. Their house was amazing. They built it in the 1970s in a simple minimalist style; it is bright and spacious and wonderfully complements their art collection. There are some seventy sculptures and more than a hundred pictures in the house – all by contemporary Czech and Moravian artists. We played golf on three consecutive days, which was some effort. The temperature was over 30 degrees centigrade; we did not have buggies and the courses were quite hilly. The highlight was a visit to Villa Tugendhat, a modernist home built between 1928 and 1930 for a wealthy Jewish industrialist. It is one of the pioneering prototypes of modern architecture in Europe and was designed by the German architect Ludwig Mies van der Rohe. One day Jirka and Hilda took us to a glassworks factory to visit their friend Professor Jaroslav Svoboda. There were some amazing pieces varying greatly in style and colour in its museum. We bought one piece, but Professor Svoboda insisted on giving it to Sheelagh as a present. So then we purchased a second piece.

From Brno we drove to Rychnov nad Kněžnou to visit my old friend Radko and Eva Vaněk. It was a nostalgic trip, as I had worked there for three years in the early 1960s. On the final day we stopped in Hradec to have a chat with Boženka and Zdeněk, Olga's relatives. They were eighty-five and ninety-five years old respectively and looked extremely good for their age.

Our last stop was Prague, where my sister arranged for us to stay in a flat a floor below hers. Her neighbour was in her cottage and had kindly agreed for us to make use of her city apartment. In the evening we took Jiřina for dinner, and an old friend Jirka Svoboda and his girlfriend Jarka joined us. It was a lovely evening to conclude a very pleasant holiday, and I felt lucky to be enjoying life so much at the age of eighty.

In September 2014 we had three weeks in Mandelieu, where Sheelagh's relative Joan Deeny visited us. We had several good golf outings with our friend Nick Kent, including one in Château Taulane in the mountains. It is a long drive but a very spectacular one, first through the mountains, then on Route Napoléon. From Mandelieu I took a short trip to Prague to attend the wedding of Jiřinka, my grand-niece. Her sister-in-law came from Canada with her family, and the occasion was very jolly.

At the end of month I went with our Tuesday golf group, Fivers, for five days' golf in Bruges. I was delighted to find myself the overall winner of our three-day competition. Early in October we had Daniel and Kate for lunch in Anson Road. Daniel was greatly surprised when after lunch I told him that someone had delivered a small present for him. We went outside, and Sean Reynolds delivered it – a new car! It was a belated reward for his outstanding results in his A-level examinations.

Sheelagh and I attended the annual meeting of the EACTS during the middle of October in Milan. I was not there much apart from the presidential address. We met friends at the council dinner, the past presidents' dinner and the presidential dinner. We also enjoyed a meal at the restaurant Don Lysander with Marcos and Mo Murtra, to which we also invited Kathy and Sharon, two of the main organizers of the association. All in all it was a very pleasant five days. We managed to include a visit to Galleria Brera and an exhibition of Chagall's work, not forgetting the magnificent Duomo.

Through the year we continued to go to Pilates classes every Monday. We also played bridge with the Chaumetons and travelled down to Parsons Green to attend Andrew Robson's bridge school.

In November I was invited by the rector of Charles University and the dean of the Medical School in Prague to receive some special awards – a gold medal from the Medical School and a silver medal from the university – having been awarded a gold medal on the 650th anniversary of the university a few years earlier. The ceremony was held in the old Gothic hall in the Karolinum, where I had been presented with my medical degree in 1958. The whole ceremony was beautifully organized, with Petr Koutecky, my friend and former colleague at the Department of Paediatric Surgery in Prague, giving a very moving speech. This was followed by a 45-minute concert by a renowned string quartet. The hall was full, with my family and many friends in attendance. Afterwards my friends from the Kardiocentrum invited Sheelagh and me to a excellent meal in a nearby Italian restaurant. It was an unforgettable day.

Christmas was spent once more in Mandelieu where we had an enjoyable lunch with our French friend Madeleine Blanchet and another with Nick and his partner Antonia.

The year 2015 started with seeing several plays at the National Theatre and continuing with bridge and Pilates. Our Swedish friends from Mandelieu, Olle and Anna Bovin, came to London. We took them to the theatre to see *Shakespeare in Love* and to Tate Modern and finished with a lovely dinner at Rules, a very traditional English restaurant off the Strand.

HOUSE RENOVATIONS AND FURTHER HOLIDAYS, 2008–2015

In February we spent two weeks in the Dominican Republic with our friends Květa and Peter Trent. Květa found a fantastic bargain: two weeks in a five-star hotel, everything – inclluding drinks and golf – for £1,000 each excluding flights. We played a lot of golf and bridge, enjoyed the beach and took a trip to San Domingo, the second largest city of the Republic. Each evening we had the dilemma of where to eat. We were spoiled for choice with very good French, Italian, Spanish, seafood and American restaurants. Two enjoyable weeks passed rather quickly.

On 1 April we were invited to Portugal, where we had five pleasant days in a house belonging to a doctor friend of Maureen's and Ajit's. We had plenty of golf, food and, in particular, drink, as is usually the case when Toni and Maureen are around. In May we had three days in Dublin visiting Sheelagh's friends from her student days. We played golf in Killiney by the sea, went to the famous Abbey Theatre and another day we had dinner with her friend Maeve. During a brief visit to Prague I managed to see an exhibition of Mucha and another of a famous Czech photographer called Saudek and of Andy Warhol.

Sheelagh's niece's husband Bryan Jenkins proposed us for country membership in Porthcawl, a very famous golf course in Wales, and one weekend we drove there, played a day with the captain and another with the president. So Sheelagh is now a member, and I have been promised membership shortly. In June we had very good three weeks in Mandelieu, discovering some new restaurants and playing more golf. Jo and Jean Barnard joined us for a few days, which was very enjoyable. We took them to St Paul de Vence and to Antibes.

In July we went for two days to Paris by Eurostar. We wanted to see the renovated and recently reopened Musée Picasso. We added a visit to Musée d'Orsay and to the Pompidou Centre. In August we embarked on another big expedition, this time to the Arctic. We flew from London to Oslo and spent the whole day exploring the city. There was a major exhibition of Van Gogh and Munch, which we found fascinating. After walking through the city, we took a boat trip around the harbour. In the evening we had an excellent dinner at Oro Bar and Grill, a highly recommended restaurant. The next day we flew to Longyearbyen, the capital of Svalbard. It was a rather bleak town. We went for lunch in a local restaurant that resembled a wooden hut. The food was very good – but to our surprise there were busts of Lenin and Marx above the bar. Apparently part of the island belongs to Russia, and old habits die hard. After a visit to the local museum and a walk around, we boarded our ship, the *Ocean Nova*, which had small but adequate cabins. The shower cubicle was minuscule, so when the boat started to rock it was not easy to take a shower. We were very pleased to see three of the team members who had been with us in the Antarctic, especially Colin, the whale specialist. We cruised through the fjords of Svalbard for four days, and we saw a polar bear with a cub, several glaciers calving, reindeer and walruses. On board we had excellent food, with a buffet at lunchtimes and sit-down dinners. Wine was inexpensive – not like Norway.

Some of the talks on board were fascinating, particularly one on Fridtjof Nansen, the Norwegian explorer and Nobel Peace Prize laureate, and another on bears. We were fascinated to learn that some birds fly non-stop from Alaska to New Zealand. From Svalbard we sailed towards Greenland. Because of a storm in the area we took a more roundabout course, going north first before turning south. Apparently this saved us a considerable amount of time. During the trip we made good friends with two New Zealand women who lived in Australia and with a Hungarian woman who was married to a Slovak. They had managed to escape from Hungary in a lorry full of potatoes, but it also took a large bribe to make sure that the soldiers at the border did not prod the potatoes too much. She subsequently went to live in Buenos Aires.

We had a contingent of Chinese and Japanese tourists on board. One Japanese woman was eighty-six years old but managed to accompany us on some fairly challenging walks. We saw musk oxen and visited interesting archaeological sites of the ancient Thule and Dorset people. We entered rather complex and deep fjords, where we had a chance to observe another polar bear. One trip out on the Zodiacs was particularly memorable. We sailed around enormous icebergs, saw numerous calvings and unusual birds. One day we woke up to a nice sunny day, surrounded completely by ice. The captain stopped for the night, because he could not see a way out of the fjord, but fortunately he managed to get moving in the morning. When asked if the ship ever got stuck in ice, he replied in the affirmative, saying that occasionally it could be stuck for several days.

A visit to an Inuit settlement was extremely interesting. There were about 400 inhabitants, living by hunting seals, polar bears and whales. There are only about 55,000 inhabitants in the whole of Greenland, which is a huge landmass. On the east coast, which we visited, there are around 5,000 people. After another two days at sea we arrived in Iceland, visiting an impressive waterfall. The last night on board we were lucky to see the Northern Lights before we arrived at Reykjavik the following morning. We hired a car and made several trips from our hotel, the Holt, including one to the Blue Lagoon, a warm swimming place where the lovely blue water is about 39 degrees centigrade. The next day we drove to the Gullfoss waterfall and Geysir hot spring. The Stokur geyser was particularly interesting, spitting a 20-metre spout every five or six minutes. On the way back to Reykjavik we stopped in Thingvellir National Park, where the American and Eurasian tectonic plates meet. They separate by about three centimetres every year, so now the gap is several kilometres, with a large lake in between. The edge of the American plate was very dramatic.

Each evening we had wonderful meals in restaurants. In Tofran – previously called the Lobster House – we had fantastic langoustines. They gave us so many that we couldn't eat them all. The Fish Market was also very good, as was the final night's venue, Perlan, a revolving restaurant on top of a hill. The food was great, but Sheelagh got food poisoning, so we were not sure whether she would be fit to fly home the next day. Fortunately she was, so we arrived back in London as scheduled, but it took her a few days to recover completely. On the whole, the trip was well worth while, although our visit to the Antarctic had been more colourful, and we had seen a greater variety of animals there.

In September I had another outing with the Tuesday morning group, this time to Honfleur in France, where we experienced beautiful countryside, good golf and excellent food. The day after our return Sheelagh and I went for three weeks to Mandelieu. Our annual EACTS meeting was in Amsterdam. Unfortunately Sheelagh had developed a bad cold, so she decided not to go. I had a very enjoyable five days, with a visit to the Rijksmuseum, the Van Gogh Museum, the Staatliche Museum, the Museum of Handbags and Rembrandt's House. I was reunited with several old friends, notably Torkel and Gunn Åberg, who had returned from Australia where they had lived for the previous seven years.

Sheelagh then took four of her girlfriends to Mandelieu, while I visited Prague. After that, I joined her in the South of France for another three weeks. This time we discovered some new restaurants in Nice and played golf in St Donat, which we had not visited for some time. They offered eighteen holes plus gourmand, an excellent two-course meal. We also went to Auribeau, a pleasant little village about twenty minutes' drive from us to have a lunch at La Table du Village, a wonderful little restaurant with exceptional food. Joan Deeny visited us for five days, which was enjoyable. At the end of our stay we organized a drinks party for Anna and Olle, Sonia and her son Axel, Danielle and Laurence. It was all very jolly.

Looking back, I feel fortunate to continue to enjoy good health and to be able to engage in my hobbies and interests and be among friends and loved ones. Sheelagh and I have continued to play golf and visit the London theatre, and we regularly attend exhibitions and filmed transmissions of operas and ballets from the Metropolitan Opera House in New York at our local cinema in Finchley. We still have enjoyable holidays at our home in Mandelieu, in the Dominican Republic and even in the Arctic. Looking back at my life and career – my family, my work and all that I have done and enjoyed – I realize my good fortune over the years. How my life would have developed if I had stayed in Prague I cannot imagine. I have come a long way since those early days in Czechoslovakia.